The Successful Occupational Therapy Fieldwork Student

The Successful Occupational Therapy Fieldwork Student

Edited by

Karen Sladyk, PhD, OTR, FAOTA

Chair of Occupational Therapy

Bay Path College

Longmeadow, Massachusetts

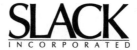

An innovative information, education and management company
6900 Grove Road • Thorofare, NJ 08086

ISBN: 978-1-55642-562-2

The procedures and practices described in this book should be implemented in a manner consistent with the professional standards set for the circumstances that apply in each specific situation. Every effort has been made to confirm the accuracy of the information presented and to correctly relate generally accepted practices. The authors, editor, and publisher cannot accept responsibility for errors or exclusions or for the outcome of the material presented herein. There is no expressed or implied warranty of this book or information imparted by it. Care has been taken to ensure that drug selection and dosages are in accordance with currently accepted/recommended practice. Due to continuing research, changes in government policy and regulations, and various effects of drug reactions and interactions, it is recommended that the reader carefully review all materials and literature provided for each drug, especially those that are new or not frequently used. Any review or mention of specific companies or products is not intended as an endorsement by the author or publisher.

SLACK Incorporated uses a review process to evaluate submitted material. Prior to publication, educators or clinicians provide important feedback on the content that we publish. We welcome feedback on this work.

Published by: SLACK Incorporated
                6900 Grove Road
                Thorofare, NJ 08086 USA
                Telephone: 856-848-1000
                Fax: 856-848-6091
                www.slackbooks.com

Contact SLACK Incorporated for more information about other books in this field or about the availability of our books from distributors outside the United States.

Library of Congress Cataloging-in-Publication Data

The successful occupational therapy fieldwork student / edited by Karen
Sladyk.
     p. ; cm.
Includes bibliographical references and index.
  ISBN 1-55642-562-7 (alk. paper)
  1. Occupational therapy–Study and teaching.
  [DNLM: 1. Occupational Therapy–education. 2. Curriculum. 3.
Internship, Nonmedical. 4. Occupational Therapy–methods. WB 18 S942
2002] I. Sladyk, Karen, 1958-
  RM735.42 .S83 2002
  615.8'515'0711–dc21
                       2002004043

Printed in the United States of America.

Last digit is print number: 10   9   8   7   6   5   4

DEDICATION

To all academic fieldwork coordinators and fieldwork educators:
At times, your exhausting work goes unnoticed.
This book is dedicated to you as a token of the profession's warm thanks.

CONTENTS

ABOUT THE EDITOR

Karen Sladyk, PhD, OTR, FAOTA, earned her OT degree from Eastern Michigan University, her MS in community health from Southern Connecticut State University, and her PhD in adult and vocational education from the University of Connecticut. Currently the chair of OT at Bay Path College in Longmeadow, MA, she is part of a faculty that offers both occupational therapy and occupational therapy assisting degrees. This fieldwork book is her eighth book with SLACK Incorporated. All her writing has been specifically designed to help students succeed in occupational therapy programs. When not busy with academic issues, Karen enjoys creative occupations, such as quilting, photography, and crafting. She volunteers at the local animal shelter. She lives in a 154-year-old house, in constant need of upkeep, with her two cats, Oliver and Laura.

Mary Alicia Barnes, OTR, received her bachelor's degree from Tufts University-Boston School for Occupational Therapy in 1985. She has been a fieldwork educator for 15 years and an academic fieldwork coordinator at Tufts University for 8 years. Her occupational therapy practice has centered on working with adolescents with severe and persistent emotional disturbance in inpatient or residential settings. She has presented and published in child and adolescent mental health, group practice, fieldwork, supervision, and professional development. When not at work, she enjoys walking, bike riding, camping, or spending time with her husband, daughter, friends, and family.

Sandy Bell, PhD, PT, is currently assistant professor in the Adult Learning program at the University of Connecticut, Storrs. She holds a PhD in adult and vocational education and an MS in physical therapy. Her research and teaching interests include adult learning and development, adaptation to injury and illness, and application of technologies to facilitate learning. Most recently, Sandy has been an invited speaker and has been published in the area of facilitating adult learning in the workplace. When not at her desk or working with students, Sandy can be found outdoors pulling weeds from her garden, getting stuck in the mud with her mountain bike, or teaching her old dog, Bean, new tricks.

Linda Duncombe, EdD, OTR, FAOTA, has been an occupational therapist for more than 33 years. She has been on the faculty at Boston University and the academic fieldwork coordinator for more than 13 years. Linda supervises level I students in community settings during the school year and level II students on mental health internships while working per-diem during the summer. She enjoys spending time at a little cabin in New Hampshire with family, friends, and nature.

Georganna Joary Miller, MEd, OTR, is academic fieldwork coordinator at Xavier University in Cincinnati, Ohio. She has experience across the specialties and supervised a large occupational therapy department for 12 years prior to her academic career. Her other occupations include wife to an IRS employee and mother to a promising teenage soccer superstar. She works in private practice, home care, and community residences. Georganna enjoys quilting, gardening, and reading.

Donna Latella, MA, OTR, is assistant academic fieldwork coordinator at Quinnipiac University in Hamden, CT, and is currently pursuing a doctoral degree in education. Her clinical background is in acute care, outpatient rehabilitation, and skilled nursing homes. Donna has recently supervised students in an adult day care center where she and her golden retriever, Cody, also volunteer, providing animal-assisted therapy to clients. Donna and Cody are a certified pet partner team through the Delta Society. Donna enjoys jogging and spending time with her husband, two children, and two dogs.

Nancy Lowenstein, MS, OTR, BCN, has spent her OT career working with adults with physical disabilities in a variety of settings including home care, long-term care, and a multiple sclerosis clinic. Nancy has taught in both technical and professional occupational therapy programs, spending many years as an academic fieldwork coordinator. She enjoys spending time with her husband, watching her sons' sport teams, and playing tennis.

Heidi McHugh Pendleton, PhD, OTR, has been an occupational therapist for more than 25 years with clinical experience in rehabilitation of adults and children with physical disabilities. During her clinical time, she welcomed the opportunity to supervise occupational therapy students. Currently, she teaches at San Jose State University in her area of expertise, having previously served a 4-year term as academic fieldwork coordinator. Heidi enjoys entertaining, cooking, reading, participating in her book club, and being with friends and family.

Beth O'Sullivan, MPH, OTR, has her master's degree in public health from the University of Connecticut and is currently the academic fieldwork coordinator at Quinnipiac University in Hamden, CT. Her clinical interests include pediatrics and neurorehabilitation. Currently, she maintains a private practice in birth to three services, consulting with parents and day care centers on developmental milestones. When not working, she remains busy with her two young daughters, who are full of energy.

Jennifer Ruisi Cosgrove, MS, OTR, is academic fieldwork coordinator at Sacred Heart University in Fairfield, CT. She received her BS in occupational therapy from Quinnipiac University, Hamden, CT, a master's degree in management from Rensselaer Polytechnic Institute, and is currently pursuing a doctoral degree in education from the University of Bridgeport. Jennifer continues to work clinically at Yale New Haven Hospital. She lives in Hamden, CT, with her husband Chris and enjoys weight training.

Winifred Schultz-Krohn, PhD, OTR, BCP, FAOTA, has more than 20 years' experience in occupational therapy. She supervised and developed fieldwork programs at a variety of clinical sites. Wynn currently teaches at San Jose State University, supervises fieldwork students at a homeless shelter, and recently received her PhD. She makes time to take walks with her husband, play with their "snottie Scottie" dog, visit family and friends, horseback ride with her niece, and quilt with her sister-in-law.

Brenda Smaga, MS, OTR, FAOTA, has a masters of science in occupational therapy from Columbia University. She is the former director of the OTA program at Manchester Community College in Connecticut. Brenda is currently the academic fieldwork coordinator at Bay Path College in Longmeadow, MA. She started her career in psychiatry and over the years has become a generalist with special interest in assistive technology. She resides in Glastonbury, CT, with her husband Mike and children, Eli and Leila.

Kathryn L. Splinter-Watkins, MOT, OTR, has been the academic fieldwork coordinator at Eastern Kentucky University in Richmond for 13 years. She currently serves as the academic fieldwork representative on the Commission on Education at AOTA, chairing the fieldwork issues committee. Her clinical interests include hippotherapy, therapeutic horseback riding, eating disorders, and pediatric mental health. She enjoys photography, playing piano, and interacting with animals, especially her cats, dog, horses, and wild birds. Kathy and her husband, Steve, enjoy working on their thoroughbred farm with their mares and foals.

Amy Lynne Thornton, MS, OTR, received her MS in occupational therapy from Tufts University-Boston School of Occupational Therapy in 2001. She is a recipient of the Association of Tufts Alumni Award for learning and leadership. Amy currently works as an occupational therapist at the New England Sinai Hospital and Rehabilitation Center in Stoughton, MA. In her free time, she enjoys exercising, spending time with friends and family, and reading about current research relevant to her practice.

Donna Whitehouse, MHA, OTR, is the academic fieldwork coordinator at Washington University in St Louis, MO. She is responsible for coordinating student level I and II clinical fieldworks, teaching professional development programs, and teaching management. Her occupational therapy practice interests include geriatric skilled nursing facilities administration and management. She enjoys working on her new home, photography, and traveling, and is currently enjoying the arrival of her newly adopted daughter from China.

JoAnne Wright, PhD, OTR, is the director of occupational therapy at the University of Utah in Salt Lake City. She attended Tufts and the University of Southern California for her PhD in occupational science with a certificate in gerontology. She and her husband, Lance, are avid travelers, rock collectors, and fossil hunters. Weekends find them fly fishing and hiking. JoAnne is a native of Utah and is glad to be back around family in the gorgeous outdoors of Utah.

PREFACE

There are many heroes in the process of becoming an occupational therapist or occupational therapy assistant. Students endure long hours of study, and educators spend hours preparing information for students to learn. Two people in this process are often the profession's greatest advocates—the academic fieldwork coordinator and the fieldwork educator. They are the two (or more) practitioners who work to help students successfully pass through the fieldwork gates.

This book was designed to help students successfully navigate the fieldwork process from level I to level II fieldwork and beyond. The book is full of true stories of successes and failures, including stories so recent the students had not even finished fieldwork when the book went to the publisher. Learning from someone else's failure is a lot easier than experiencing it yourself.

Although all fieldwork experiences are included in this book, the reader will notice a focus on level II fieldwork. Typically, students have more support during level I fieldwork and are more independent at level II. This book is full of stories and activities to help support the more independent experience and prepare the future practitioner for entry-level practice.

First, a few notes for the reader. Although this book has 16 fieldwork experts as authors, only your academic fieldwork coordinator understands your unique needs. Always consult with your school's faculty before making fieldwork decisions that may impact your success.

Writing a book is never an easy task. It is a team experience from idea generation to bookstore shelf. There are many people to thank. First to my gifted contributing authors who warmly accepted their challenges while making room in their other "occupations" to write for this book. Thanks to their friends and family members who supported them and proofread for us. A special thanks goes to the people at SLACK Incorporated, especially Amy McShane, who has become a dear friend. Thank you to Debra Toulson and April Johnson for making our work look so great. Last, I thank the faculty and students who use this book as part of their fieldwork success.

Karen Sladyk, PhD, OTR, FAOTA

Section I

INTRODUCTION

Chapter 1

Purpose and Process of Fieldwork

Karen Sladyk, PhD, OTR, FAOTA

No matter what college or university you are enrolled in as an OT or OTA student, you will participate in fieldwork experiences as part of your curriculum. The American Occupational Therapy Association (AOTA) has a division that oversees occupational therapy curricula nationwide. The Accreditation Council for Occupational Therapy Education (ACOTE) has developed minimum standards that all OT and OTA programs must meet to be accredited, and these standards include fieldwork (ACOTE, 1998). Because accreditation is required for a student to be able to take the certification exam to practice, every occupational therapy curriculum in the nation and some overseas participate in fieldwork.

Fieldwork is the beginning of a lifelong learning experience. This book is a collection of writings from some of the leading experts in fieldwork education in the United States. The purpose of this book is to take readers from the planning stage through fieldwork to supervising their own fieldwork students. Information is presented in a comfortable reading style with numerous activities and stories to encourage student reflection. When possible, authors were asked to provide true stories from real fieldwork experiences. Although readers may think they see themselves or others in these stories, the truth is that the stories are typical of many students. Our hope is that future fieldwork students can learn from the activities and stories in this book.

The book begins with an overview of the purpose and process of fieldwork. By the end of this chapter, you should understand the following:

➡ The language of fieldwork.

➡ The goals of level I and II fieldwork.

➡ The special demands of fieldwork.

➡ The role of attitude in successful fieldwork.

LANGUAGE OF FIELDWORK

Before we can begin to address the details of the fieldwork experience, it is helpful to understand the language used. Fieldwork is divided into two levels: I and II. Note that the one and two are always written as Roman numerals. Level I fieldwork is typically in conjunction with classroom activities, and level II fieldwork is typically done after classes are completed. ACOTE provides schools with some flexibility to design level I fieldwork so that the experience can closely match the school's specific curriculum design. Level II fieldwork, however, has minimum requirements such as time, supervision, and type of experiences. Generally, the goal of level I fieldwork is to have experiences with people with and without disabilities, while the goal of level II fieldwork is to demonstrate entry-level skills as an occupational therapy practitioner.

Level I Fieldwork

ACOTE (1998) describes level I fieldwork as integrated into the curriculum designed to enrich classroom material including observation and participation in selected aspects of the occupational therapy process. The focus is not independent performance. It is important for students to understand that the goal of level I fieldwork is not necessarily to get you ready for level II fieldwork. Although the fieldworks are numbered chronologically, the goals of the fieldworks are very different. Level I fieldwork may be observational only or may include limited opportunities for students to practice a specific skill, often in pairs. Level I fieldwork may have occupational therapy personnel as supervisors or may have other disciplines, such as nursing, social work, recreation, education, or case management. Level I fieldwork may be in medical model sites, such as hospitals or rehabilitation clinics, but is more likely to be in community model sites such as schools, assistive living centers, and summer camp programs.

Level II Fieldwork

ACOTE (1998) describes level II fieldwork's goal to develop competent entry-level practitioners. Because level II fieldwork is more complex than level I, each person involved in the experience may have different goals in mind. The school's goal may be for the student to apply theory to practice. The site's goal may be for the student to demonstrate entry-level practice. The student's goal may be to learn hands-on with real consumers.

Academic Fieldwork Coordinator

Although this name may be different in each school, the academic fieldwork coordinator (AFWC) is the person(s) assigned by the college or university to oversee the fieldwork program. This person may specifically address level II fieldwork or may have responsibilities in level I, II, and prefieldwork experiences including service learning programs. The AFWC is the expert in the fieldwork process and should be the first person a student sees on campus if he or she has questions concerning fieldwork. The very first step a student should take is to fill out Appendix A. Update and keep this information handy from today through your professional career.

Fieldwork Educator

This person is sometimes called the clinical educator depending on the site. On level II fieldwork, the fieldwork educator (FE) is the occupational therapy practitioner who supervises the student at the specific site. The FE for level I fieldwork may be from another discipline. While on fieldwork, the student should address all questions to the FE before bringing questions to other staff or back to the school.

Traditional Practice Areas

Students often imagine themselves working in traditional practice areas such as rehabilitation clinics and school systems. Occupational therapy has a long history in physical and psychiatric hospitals as well as nursing homes and, more recently, school systems and private practice. These areas will continue to employ OTs and OTAs, but funding in these areas has recently been dramatically reduced.

Emerging Practice Areas

Different from traditional sites, emerging areas offer the OT and OTA exciting challenges to develop new practice arenas, such as rural practice, home care, community wellness centers, assistive living centers, summer camps, community clubhouse programs, and halfway houses. These sites offer excellent opportunities for program development but also require mature, flexible, and adaptive students. As reduced funding in traditional practice areas continues, occupational therapy's growth will continue in emerging areas.

DEMANDS AFFECTING FIELDWORK

Family ▶
Demands ▶

College Student
▼▼▼

◀ Work
◀ Demands

Financial ▶
Demands ▶

Fieldwork Student
▼▼▼

◀ Crisis
◀ Management

Study Time ▶
Demands ▶

Exam Candidate
▼▼▼

◀ Anxiety Over The Exam

Practitioner

ISSUES OF REIMBURSEMENT AFFECTING FIELDWORK

Students enter the profession of occupational therapy because they enjoy helping people find meaning in their occupations. Unfortunately, the role of money often interferes with this process. Reimbursement in health care has been a major issue in the United States for the past 20 years. In the early 1990s, occupational therapy saw a huge growth in jobs and salaries as for-profit companies saw great profits in billing for both occupational and physical therapy services. Congress saw this and other price gouging in medicine and put in place the Balanced Budget Act of 1997, resulting in decreased reimbursement for almost all medical services. The results were dramatic, with staff being laid off and students unable to find fieldwork placements in traditional sites.

Other rules have also limited some fieldwork sites from accepting fieldwork students. These include staffing patterns, Medicare rules on supervision, and third-party payers. Despite these radical changes in health care, occupational therapy has rebounded and is growing in emerging practice areas. Students are finding jobs with less difficulty, and employers are reporting greater staff openings as they grow out of the reimbursement problems of the past.

A related issue to reimbursement is often asked by students: "If I'm providing services for the site to bill, how come I'm not getting a stipend and why am I paying tuition?" The answers to these questions are multilevel. Most schools charge tuition for fieldwork because college credit is awarded. The AFWC position is often a full-time position that requires specialized training and expertise. Tuition revenue often helps pay to recruit and retain this expert. Developing fieldwork sites requires other expenditures, such as legal aid for contract review, fieldwork site visits, clerical support, malpractice insurance, and fieldwork educator support. Tuition helps cover these costs.

As for providing treatment services from which the site is generating revenue, most of the research on cost analysis of fieldwork students shows an even wash of expenditures and revenues during fieldwork (Meyers, 1995; Shalik, 1987; Shalik & Shalik, 1988). Detailed reviews have suggested that fieldwork sites lose revenue during a student's first level II fieldwork and only slightly financially benefit if the student is on his or her second level II fieldwork site. Because fieldwork sites typically lose revenue by accepting fieldwork students, stipends would further affect revenue and are rarely offered.

DEMANDS OF FIELDWORK

Each school and fieldwork site has expectations for successful completion of fieldwork. These vary greatly from program to program, so finding the "just right challenge" is a challenge in itself. Level I fieldwork is likely very structured to meet the academic program's expectation. Level II fieldwork likely has two sets of expectations, the school's and the fieldwork sites'. No doubt you will have expectations yourself. In addition to being a fieldwork student, you likely have other demands. Because level II fieldwork is full-time, maintaining an additional job often interferes with fieldwork performance, and this financial issue is often a problem for students.

If you truly understand the role of occupation in people's lives, then you have analyzed your own occupations and personal goals. Likely, a personal goal is to become an occupational therapy practitioner. This includes a process of completing several milestones (see *Demands Affecting Fieldwork*). Although a linear process in theory, we know from our study of occupation that many obstacles interfere with our milestones. This book is designed to help students, beginning in school through entry-level practice, be successful. We begin by briefly looking at what makes a successful fieldwork student. All of these attributes will be discussed further throughout this book.

ATTITUDE MAKES ALL THE DIFFERENCE

As an educator for more than 10 years of both OTs and OTAs, I can share my experience in successful fieldwork. As an AFWC for nearly 5 years, I traveled the United States providing program supervision to hundreds of students and fieldwork sites. The clear issue that separated most successful students from most unsuccessful students was attitude. Attitude is difficult to define because many people believe they have a positive attitude while others see them as self-centered, closed to supervision, even pig-headed. Successful students were open to continual feedback, seeing opportunities for growth instead of moments of personal judgment. Even students who, in theory, were not ready for fieldwork because of academic issues were successful because they wanted personal and professional growth, despite being exhausted by extra work, to understand clinical experiences.

As an example of how attitude can make a difference in fieldwork success, I direct your attention back to your childhood. No matter how old you are, you may remember a childhood magazine called *Highlights for Children*. It seemed this magazine was always popular in the dentist's waiting room and included a section called Goofus and Gallant. Goofus was a child with an attitude while Gallant always did things positively. Goofus was always rude and had a sour look on his face while Gallant looked happy and eager to please. Fieldwork can draw from this childhood example, and true OT fieldwork stories are listed under Goofus in *True Fieldwork Stories* (p. 7).

The first example in True Fieldwork Stories is a classic story reported by almost every AFWC. A student tells her supervisor, "I'm not really interested in this practice area." What the supervisor hears the student say is, "I'm not very interested in the practice area that you have chosen for your life's work. I'll just do the minimum I need to get through because I have to be here." As an occupational therapy educator, I have spent time educating students about how this appears rude, but, year after year, a fieldwork supervisor reports a student making this statement. Keep in mind

that everything you say to any occupational therapy practitioner is important, as the OT world is small and burnt bridges are hard to mend.

A review of the literature on fieldwork success shows fieldwork educators are less concerned with student skills than attitude (Ellis, 2000; Herzberg, 1994; Kautzmann, 1987; Kramer & Stern, 1995; Sladyk & Sheckley, 1999). *Positive Attributes* (p. 8) lists the attributes clinicians believe are important to a successful fieldwork experience. When you look at the whole list, you can see how the role of attitude is important. It sets the right mood, and it makes relationships go more smoothly. Your AFWC may ask you to write him or her a letter or journal entry describing how you typically show these attributes.

SUMMARY

So how can you make sure you have a positive attitude for fieldwork? That's what this book is for. Experts in fieldwork from around the country were invited to participate in the development of this book. Together, the authors of this book have hundreds of years of experience with FEs. They not only have been AFWCs, but also FEs as well. They are writing to share their true stories of successful and less successful fieldwork experiences.

REFERENCES

Accreditation Council for Occupational Therapy Education. (1998). *Standards for an accredited educational program for the occupational therapist (occupational therapy assistant)*. Bethesda, MD: American Occupational Therapy Association.

Ellis, D. (2000). *Becoming a master student*. Boston, MA: Houghton Mifflin Company.

Herzberg, G. L. (1994). The successful fieldwork student: Supervisor perceptions. *Am J Occup Ther, 48*(9), 817-823.

Kautzmann, L. (1987). Perceptions of the purpose of level I fieldwork. *Am J Occup Ther, 41*(9), 595-600.

Kramer, P., & Stern, K. (1995). Approaches to improving student performance on fieldwork. *Am J Occup Ther, 49*(2), 156-159.

Meyers, S. K. (1995). Exploring the costs and benefits drivers of clinical education. *Am J Occup Ther, 49*(2), 107-111.

Shalik, L. D. (1987). Cost benefit analysis of level II fieldwork in occupational therapy. *Am J Occup Ther, 41*(10), 638-645.

TRUE FIELDWORK STORIES

	Goofus type	*Gallant type*
During the initial meeting with the student, the supervisor asks about his or her interests in this specialty. The student honestly does not have an interest in the supervisor's specialty.	The student responds, "I'm not interested in this area, but my school requires I have a fieldwork here."	The student responds, "I'm open-minded and have not made any final decisions about my practice interests yet."
During the interview for a possible placement, the supervisor ends the overview by asking if the student has any questions.	The student responds, "You covered everything well but what about lunch and parking?"	The student responds, "You covered everything well, but could you tell me a little more about the theories the staff use in assessment and treatment?"
At midterm, the supervisor tells the student he or she is below expectations.	The student responds, "You never said this before. You said I did well with today's patient, maybe you should rethink the evaluation."	The student responds, "I hear your concerns and I would like to think about them. Can I set up an appointment with you for later this afternoon?"
The supervisor is touring the AFWC around the clinic when they enter the office area. The student has his or her feet up on the desk. The supervisor seems embarrassed. The AFWC says, "Remove your feet."	The student responds, "We are very informal here."	The student does not put his or her feet on the desk.
The supervisor asks the student not to wear a particular outfit again.	The student responds, "Why? This is very fashionable and I saw other staff wearing the same thing."	The student responds, "Of course. Would you like me to go home, change, and return during lunch?"
The student accepts a scholarship for a conference paid for by the department but then misses 1 of the 2 days because of a prior commitment.	The student offers no explanation.	The student investigates prior commitments and declines the scholarship in favor of someone who can use both days.
The supervisor is 5 minutes late to a meeting.	The student responds, "Where have you been?"	The student does not call attention to the time.
The site has determined that the student has failed the fieldwork experience. The supervisor tells the student at the end of the day and asks the student to meet with him or her and the AFWC first thing tomorrow.	The student responds, "This is not fair. I'm doing as well as the other students. I want to file a complaint. I'm going to notify the school and the other students of discrimination."	The student responds, "I do not know what to say. May I call my AFWC before I leave today?"

POSITIVE ATTRIBUTES

➠ Show interest in the specialty and the profession
➠ Take responsibility for your attitude
➠ Separate liking from learning
➠ Seek additional information
➠ Avoid excuses
➠ Submit professional work on time
➠ Arrive a bit early to organize your day
➠ Accept criticism
➠ Use supervision time effectively
➠ Take on new projects
➠ Provide feedback to supervisors
➠ Keep up on problems and ideas
➠ Listen
➠ Practice
➠ Manage time
➠ Care about the consumer's issues
➠ Remember safety first
➠ Be creative in solving problems

Adapted from Sladyk, K., & Sheckley, B. (1999). Differences between clinical reasoning gainers and decliners during fieldwork. In *Innovations in occupational therapy education.* Bethesda, MD: American Occupational Therapy Association and Ellis, D. (2000). *Becoming a master student.* Boston, MA: Houghton Mifflin Company.

Shalik, H., & Shalik, L. D. (1988). The occupational therapy level II fieldwork experience: Estimation of the fiscal benefit. *Am J Occup Ther, 42*(3), 164-168.

Sladyk, K., & Sheckley, B. (1999). Differences between clinical reasoning gainers and decliners during fieldwork. In *Innovations in occupational therapy education.* Bethesda, MD: American Occupational Therapy Association.

Note: Highlights for Children *is published by Highlights for Children, Inc., 1800 Watermark Drive, PO Box 269, Columbus, OH 43216-0269.*

Chapter 2

Learning Objectives for the Fieldwork Experience

Winifred Schultz-Krohn, PhD, OTR, BCP, FAOTA
Heidi McHugh Pendleton, PhD, OTR

The purpose of the fieldwork experience is to provide you, the student, with an opportunity to integrate and apply your academic knowledge and skills to progressively more demanding levels of performance and responsibility (American Occupational Therapy Association [AOTA], 1996; Cohn, 1989).

At the completion of this chapter and the guided exercises, you will be able to do the following:

➡ Identify, define, and apply the components of a learning objective.

➡ Understand the importance of learning objectives for completion of the fieldwork experience.

➡ Relate a learning objective at a specific fieldwork site to the Fieldwork Evaluation Form (FWEF).

➡ Understand the importance and developmental nature of the clinical reasoning process and its relationship to meeting the fieldwork objectives.

➡ Identify strategies to meet student fieldwork objectives.

➡ Recognize the progressive nature and increasing demands of fieldwork objectives during the fieldwork experience.

In order to accomplish entry-level competency, each fieldwork site customarily develops and lists a series of fieldwork objectives, often predicated on the experiences of previous fieldwork students at the site. These objectives are ordinarily arranged in weekly increments with the goals of subsequent weeks building upon the objectives of the previous weeks. Your job, as a fieldwork student, is to become informed regarding the objectives of the specific fieldwork site and determine how you will meet each of these objectives with the ultimate goal of entry-level competency at the end of the fieldwork experience.

One approach you might take—which is the model used for this chapter—is to consider that the fieldwork site student objectives are similar to the process one uses for developing and carrying out a patient treatment plan. In this case, you are both the patient and practitioner, the treatment plan is the internship process, and the outcome is the successful completion of the fieldwork experience. The chapter begins by defining what is meant by an objective with examples of student objectives from a variety of fieldwork sites, and then identifies how the fieldwork objective is linked with the AOTA FWEF, both for the OT and the OTA student. Next, suggestions or strategies are offered for meeting the fieldwork objectives, including use of clinical reasoning and use of environmental supports. The chapter concludes with guided exercises to practice using the newly learned approaches for meeting the fieldwork objectives.

STUDENT LEARNING OBJECTIVES

What are student learning objectives at a fieldwork site? They are specific behaviors that a student must exhibit to successfully complete the fieldwork experience (Kramer & Stern, 1995). These objectives range from familiarizing yourself with the fieldwork setting to performing client treatment sessions with appropriate documentation and assuming responsibility for professional behavior at the fieldwork site.

Why are learning objectives important to the fieldwork experience? Clearly stated learning objectives provide a target for the student to measure his or her performance against the expectations of the fieldwork site. Learning objectives also allow the occupational therapy student to chart progress of his or her own skills over the course of the fieldwork experience.

A learning objective for a specific fieldwork experience should closely resemble a client objective or goal. A well-written objective consists of three parts (Pedretti & Early, 2001; Zimmerman, 1988):

1. A behavioral statement or targeted behavior that identifies what is expected of the student.

2. A measure or criterion statement that identifies the level of performance expected of the student.

3. A condition statement that identifies the environmental circumstances, including the resources or strategies, that must be in place for the stated behavior to occur.

An example of a fieldwork objective that possesses all three components is, "Using newly learned test administration strategies, the student will independently administer the Peabody Developmental Motor Scales to one child."

The *behavioral* statement is "administer the Peabody Developmental Motor Scales to one child" (Folio & Fewell, 2000).

The *criterion* statement or measure of the student skill is "independently."

The *condition* statement is "Using newly learned test administration strategies."

Fieldwork objectives should provide a clear target behavior and criterion statement. The condition statement is not necessarily included in each student objective but, rather, may be written as a preceding experience at the fieldwork site. For example, at a different fieldwork site, a similar student objective may be written as follows: "By week 10 of the fieldwork experience, the student will independently administer the Peabody Developmental Motor Scales to one child."

In this situation, the fieldwork schedule may indicate that the student will "observe the Peabody Developmental Motor Scales administered by the clinical instructor" and "study the corresponding administration manual" during weeks 7, 8, and 9 before the expectation is made for the student to independently administer this instrument. The condition (newly learned test administration strategies) is still present and is included in the actual fieldwork schedule but is not formally stated in the student objective.

How a student will achieve the stated objective constitutes the methods or intervention portion of his or her individual student treatment/learning plan. Students must examine the learning resources available to assist them in meeting the specified objective. These learning resources include activities such as reviewing the student fieldwork manual, discussing with supervisor and staff at the fieldwork site, observing therapy sessions, reviewing previous coursework and textbooks, communicating with faculty, and engaging in library searches. This list is not meant to be exhaustive but merely to provide suggestions to the student. These methods will require the student to engage in self-directed and self-initiated learning behavior to meet the objectives. Active experimentation, adaptability, flexibility, and teamwork have been identified as characteristics of a successful fieldwork student (Herzberg, 1994). Additional resources will be discussed in a later section of this chapter.

As a student reviews the objectives for the entire fieldwork experience, he or she will notice an increasing demand on student performance as the experience progresses (Cohn, 1989). This is often seen with the number of client treatment sessions and progress notes assigned to the student. Initially, the student may only be required to write one client progress note during the first 1 to 2 weeks of the fieldwork experience. As the fieldwork experience progresses, the student is expected to be responsible for an increasing number of client notes. The overarching goal of a fieldwork experience is to help a student develop entry-level practice skills (AOTA, 1996; Kramer & Stern, 1995; Sands, 1995). To meet this goal, the fieldwork experience is designed to provide increasing responsibilities for the student.

EXAMPLES OF TYPICAL STUDENT OBJECTIVES

Following an extensive review of the fieldwork objectives from numerous sites, a similarity in the progression of student responsibilities was noted. We found that student objectives at the beginning of the fieldwork typically address the responsibility of the student to become familiar with the facility, equipment and assessments used at the site, client characteristics, schedule of meetings, and basic treatment approaches. This requires the student to become oriented to the procedures and processes used for client treatment. A student may be assigned only one or two clients initially, and ideally these clients have similar diagnostic or functional characteristics. This similarity and opportunity for repetition allows the student to begin to develop a repertoire of basic treatment skills (Cohn, 1989).

The initial objectives of the fieldwork experience must be met before the student is able to accept increasing responsibilities of later objectives. For example, a student must be familiar with the facility procedures for conducting a cooking class, such as ordering the food, checking on client dietary restrictions, and safe storage of food before the student is able to independently conduct the group.

Examples of student objectives characteristic of the initial portion of the fieldwork experience were collected from several sites. Occupational therapists from the Santa Cruz County Mental Health and Substance Abuse Center (SCCMH) shared their fieldwork objectives for occupational therapy students. During the first week, a student was expected to "look through the OT supplies closet, make a list of three items, and how you might use those items in a treatment session."

At another community-based mental health center called Community Connection in California, the student learning objective stated that during the second week of the fieldwork experience the student would "identify the common features of the clients who are diagnosed with acute depression, paranoia, schizophrenia, organic problems, and discuss those features during the supervision meeting."

At Craig Hospital, an objective for the first week of the fieldwork experience states that the student will "attend rounds, department meetings, behavior meetings, and case meetings."

Mastery of these initial objectives serves a very important purpose. The student is now oriented to the fieldwork site as well as the basic client intervention provided at the site. Accomplishing these basic goals allows the student to move into more demanding roles that are characteristic of the middle portion of the fieldwork experience. The student no longer has to expend energy to remember where reachers are stored, what form is used to record client appointments, or the common features of his or her clients' diagnoses. Energy is more appropriately allocated to the increasing number of client contact hours, the variety of clients, and the demands for documentation expected of the student. A

student who has not successfully become oriented to the fieldwork site is likely to feel overwhelmed and lost as the experience progresses.

During the middle portion of the fieldwork experience, objectives reflect the breadth of skill development relevant to that specific fieldwork setting. Objectives may require a student to work with a greater variety of clients or use a greater variety of treatment approaches. There is more than merely an increase in client contact hours noted during the middle portion of the fieldwork experience. There is also a corresponding expectation that students will demonstrate more highly sophisticated levels of problem-solving skills along with insightful documentation (Schwartz, 1984). Students should now be able to analyze and document client behavior and develop a plan to address the client's needs.

Student objectives from Rancho Los Amigos National Rehabilitation Center (RLANRC) in California provide examples that are typical of this portion of the fieldwork experience:

➡ "Caseload now consists of 4 to 5 patients (6 hours of treatment per day) with close supervision."

➡ "Treatment planning and problem solving is now initiated on own for routine patients, seeking supervision input assertively and as needed."

The fieldwork objectives from the Visiting Nurse Alliance of Vermont/New Hampshire (VNA) also demonstrate the increasing level of responsibility expected of the student. This is reflected in the following statement that during the middle portion of the affiliation the student will "independently develop home programs for clients that integrate treatment objectives."

During the final weeks of the fieldwork experience, the occupational therapy student is expected to function as an entry-level practitioner. This includes interacting with other professionals and clients. Student objectives focus on independent skills such as reporting in team meetings, client rounds, and participation at the fieldwork site. Examples of this level of responsibility are found in the following student objectives from RLANRC, the San Jose Family Shelter (SJFS), the VNA of VT/NH, and the El Dorado Center (EDC):

➡ "Establish self as integrated member of the team, primary contact person in OT for assigned patients, integrating patient's preferences into team treatment planning, and serving as a resource of information to the patient" (RLANRC).

➡ "Present inservice to staff addressing selected topic as approved by supervisor" (SJFS).

➡ "Train home health aide in specific activities of daily living program for a client" (VNA).

➡ "Participate in team meetings by reporting client data and progress" (EDC).

Relationship Between Learning Objectives and the Fieldwork Evaluation Form

The fieldwork student objectives provide systematic and specific targeted behaviors that progress the student toward successfully meeting the requirements articulated in the FWEF for both the OT (AOTA, 1987) and the OTA (AOTA, 1983) student. The FWEF provides general statements of student performance in various categories. The OTA FWEF assesses student performance in the areas of evaluation, treatment, communication, and professional behavior (AOTA, 1983). The OT FWEF looks at similar student abilities in the areas of assessment, planning, treatment, problem solving, and administration/professionalism (AOTA, 1987). These general statements identify the behaviors necessary for entry-level practice skills for both levels of occupational therapy practitioners. Student fieldwork objectives provide the specific details of how the FWEF requirements are applied to the particular fieldwork site. An example from the FWEF for the OTA student asks, "Does student correctly administer assigned evaluation procedures to obtain information relevant to client performance?" (AOTA, 1983).

The supervisor then rates the student's performance using a scale ranging from incorrect administration of evaluation procedures to exceptional ability of the student to correctly administer the evaluation tool. The fieldwork student objective for the site would identify the specific assigned evaluation tool for that site. An example of a student fieldwork learning objective that specifically articulates the expectations for this general statement would be the following: "The OTA student will correctly administer the Kohlman Evaluation of Living Skills (KELS) as directed by supervisor."

In the above example, the OTA student's ability to correctly administer the KELS (Kohlman-Thomas, 1992) to obtain information on client performance will be used by the clinical supervisor to score the corresponding FWEF item at the completion of the fieldwork experience. This provides an illustration of how the fieldwork objectives are linked to the FWEF for the OTA student.

A similar example can be seen using the FWEF for an OT student (AOTA, 1987). This form provides general statements addressing the entry-level skills necessary for the OT. One item from this form requires that the student "administers the assessment procedures according to standardized or recommended techniques" (AOTA, 1987).

The clinical supervisor would then rate the OT student's performance, judgment, and attitude with regards to the administration of an assessment. A pediatric fieldwork site may apply this general statement to the setting by writing the following student objective: "Using newly learned test administration strategies, the student will independently administer the Peabody Developmental Motor Scales to one child."

Again, the linkage is seen between the student objectives at the specific fieldwork site and the FWEF. The administration of the Peabody Developmental Motor Scales provides the OT student with the opportunity to demonstrate the ability to use standardized or recommended techniques.

Not all student fieldwork objectives have a direct or obvious application to the items on the FWEF. The objective characteristic of the first 1 or 2 weeks of the fieldwork experience typically focuses on the student becoming oriented to the site, procedures, and client population. These objectives do not have a direct relationship to the FWEF but still serve an important function. The initial objectives allow the student to become better organized to meet the increasing demands of the fieldwork experience and to achieve the basic skills needed to successfully demonstrate the behaviors expected on the FWEF. Indirectly, those initial objectives can influence student behaviors for FWEF items such as the effective use of time, compliance with institutional policies and procedures, and professional behavior by developing a foundation upon which to build and strengthen these higher level skills.

Recognizing the importance of the fieldwork objectives and their relevance to meeting the items on the FWEF for both the OT and OTA is a crucial first step toward successful completion of your fieldwork experience. In the next section, we will explore resources and strategies for successfully achieving these objectives.

How to Meet Fieldwork Objectives

There are undoubtedly countless methods and strategies you could employ for meeting the fieldwork objectives. In fact, as your fieldwork experience progresses, you will probably have your own list of successful and not-so-successful interventions that, in time, you may pass down to your own fieldwork students. In the meantime, we offer some tried-and-true suggestions learned from our own personal fieldwork experiences as well as those from many of our former fieldwork students who graciously contributed their own words of wisdom.

Any discussion of strategies for meeting student learning objectives presumes that the student has a foundation for understanding how to use clinical reasoning skills—a critical component for success as an occupational therapist or occupational therapy assistant. This section will therefore address a primary strategy for meeting student fieldwork objectives, that is, the use of clinical reasoning skills, followed by a discussion of additional strategies using environmental supports to successfully meet fieldwork objectives.

Use of Clinical Reasoning Skills to Meet Fieldwork Objectives

Clinical reasoning skills provide a framework for students to examine how they will approach fieldwork objectives (Buchanan, Moore, & van Niekerk, 1998; Neistadt, 1996; Schwartz, 1991). Cohn (1989) describes clinical reasoning as a process, dependent upon experience, in which the practitioner combines the "knowledge of procedures, interactions with patients, and interpretation and analysis of the evolving situation" (p. 241). The process of developing clinical reasoning skills has been described as following a progression from novice to expert (Neistadt, 1996; Slater & Cohn, 1991). All levels are presented here to provide the student with an understanding of the progressive nature of clinical reasoning skills even though only the novice and advanced beginner stages are considered appropriate for occupational therapy students (Neistadt, 1996).

The novice is described as rule bound, having a relatively rigid approach regarding client assessments and intervention (Slater & Cohn, 1991). A student at this level would approach fieldwork learning objectives from a perspective of completing the objective without examining the reason the objective is present at that site. The advanced beginner, in comparison, displays more flexibility for specific situations and can modify rules and procedures (Neistadt, 1996). A student functioning at this level would view the fieldwork objectives as a guide toward practice at that specific fieldwork site but may still have difficulty seeing the linkage between the fieldwork objectives and overall entry-level practice skills.

The competent level of performance is not considered to be entry level but is said to emerge after a few years of clinical practice. This level of performance is characterized by a practitioner who is able to identify the importance of various pieces of client information but who may have problems modifying intervention plans quickly in response to client needs. Neistadt (1996) states that it is not reasonable to expect occupational therapy students to graduate at the competent, proficient, or expert level of practice, but argues that students should be informed of the progressive nature of clinical reasoning skills to foster growth and development of these skills. The proficient therapist is able to alter plans easily to meet the client's needs and has an understanding of the client's total situation. The expert therapist is able to organize the "treatment more from the client's cues than from a preconceived plan of therapeutic action" (p. 677).

Neistadt (1996) identifies five types of clinical reasoning used in occupational therapy practice: *narrative reasoning*, *interactive reasoning*, *procedural reasoning*, *pragmatic reasoning*, and *conditional reasoning*. The various types of clinical reasoning allow the student to view the client from several perspectives. All forms of clinical reasoning should be employed by the student to successfully complete the fieldwork experience and operate as an entry-level practitioner.

Narrative reasoning is focused on the client's story and how the disabling condition has affected the client's occupational behavior (Clark, 1993; Mattingly, 1991). The student would use this form of reasoning to determine what activities were important to the client before the illness or injury and what the client would choose as priorities in the future. For example, not all clients have self-dressing skills as a priority. The energy expenditure to complete self-dressing tasks may not be worth the reward of independence in this skill. An occupational therapy student would use narrative reasoning to meet a fieldwork objective that states, "The student will consistently establish treatment goals with the client and family."

Interactive reasoning addresses the disability experience of the client (Crepeau, 1991; Fleming, 1991). This form of reasoning can also be viewed as the therapeutic relationship established between the therapist and the client. The student recognizes the unique perspective of the client relative to the disabling condition. The student would use interactive reasoning to meet a fieldwork objective that requires, "The student will effectively design intervention plans for a variety of clients with different mental health diagnoses."

Procedural reasoning is focused on the selection and use of appropriate assessment and intervention methods for a specific client (Fleming, 1991; Hasselkus & Dickie, 1994). The student uses this form of reasoning to meet the following fieldwork objective: Administers the KELS according to assessment instrument protocol.

Pragmatic reasoning is focused on the environmental context, including the student's skills and knowledge, the client's insurance coverage, and the support systems for the client (Creighton, Dijkers, Bennett, & Brown, 1995). This requires that the therapist understand the potential of the client and options available to the client. At the initial assessment session, the occupational therapist should begin planning for the discharge of the client. A student would engage in pragmatic reasoning to meet the following objective: Develop an appropriate discharge plan with referrals to necessary support services such as Meals on Wheels or an adult day support program for a client with impaired cognitive abilities.

Conditional reasoning requires the practitioner to engage in ongoing revisions of the treatment plan to meet the unique needs of the client (Fleming, 1991; Hasselkus & Dickie, 1994). An example would be the flexibility of the student to modify a treatment plan when faced with a client who refuses to participate in the planned activity. This ability to "think on your feet" is not merely creative problem solving but also considers the views of the client and why the client has refused to participate in the planned activity. A student would use conditional reasoning to meet a fieldwork objective that states that the student will "establish self as integrated member of the team, primary contact person in OT for assigned patients, integrating patient's preferences into team treatment planning, and serving as a resource of information to the patient" (RLANRC, Sept. 2000).

Clinical reasoning skills provide a framework to understand the importance of the fieldwork objectives. As you review the fieldwork objectives for your site, try to match the objective with the type of clinical reasoning skills you will need to meet that objective. Then, consider the resources you can use to meet that objective. Some suggestions for such resources are offered in the next section.

Use of Environmental Supports

On the first day of your fieldwork experience, it is customary to be given a copy of the site's student learning objectives arranged in order of expectations from the initial to final weeks. It will be important that you study these objectives and the FWEF to obtain an overall perspective of what will be expected of you during the fieldwork experience. You may then choose to organize and merge both the site's weekly objectives and your "newly learned" strategies for achieving those objectives into your own schedule. It is advisable to review the student learning objectives with your supervisor early in the fieldwork experience so that you can clarify any questions and discover any variations

or additional expectations your supervisor might have. Such proactive behavior is often regarded as an indication that you are taking the fieldwork seriously, are a self-starter, and are someone who is resourceful—someone who explores possible answers first and then seeks the assistance of the person with the expertise.

STRATEGIES FOR THE FIRST WEEKS OF FIELDWORK

As was indicated earlier in this chapter, the first few weeks of fieldwork are consumed with learning about the physical and procedural aspects of the fieldwork site as well as the basics regarding the diagnoses or features of the clients treated by occupational therapy at the site. Strategies are presented here addressing three categories: *orientation to the fieldwork site*, *orientation to clients and procedures*, and *orientation to documentation*.

Orient Yourself to the Fieldwork Site

If possible, take a tour of the fieldwork site prior to your first day. Correspond with your student supervisor to introduce yourself and ask questions regarding student working hours, dress code, parking, public transportation, etc., anything that you think would help make you feel comfortable regarding your first day's expectations. Record such information in a small journal that you can carry in your pocket for quick reference later. As you read the other ideas for strategies in this section, consider additional options for pertinent journal entries.

Visit the site's web site if applicable and download a map and read about the mission of the site, its history, or any other pertinent information that might help to orient you.

Some students have been known to make a trial run to the fieldwork site prior to their first day to determine the travel time, traffic patterns, and parking realities so that they are more confident about making a good first impression. Be sure that the conditions approximate those that will be in place on your first day.

Ask to see the student fieldwork manual. The majority of fieldwork sites keep a reference manual for students to use for answers to frequently asked questions. Often, the student fieldwork objectives are listed there along with safety protocols, department procedures, documentation samples, and the facility's rules and regulations. Some fieldwork manuals contain projects completed by previous fieldwork students that were added because of their relevance to future students' information needs or as exemplars of projects to inspire future students. If your fieldwork site does not have a student manual, you might want to start one for your own use and then later offer it to the site for the benefit of future students. This is frequently the way fieldwork manuals come into being or are updated.

To learn where things are in the OT clinic/treatment area, come early or use part of your lunch break to clean out an equipment closet. This allows you to learn what items are available, become familiar with novel items, and develop ideas for treatment. The more familiar and comfortable you feel with where things are located, the more likely you will be able to focus on the higher level and more creative aspects of client treatment.

Orient Yourself to Clients and Procedures

Review class notes and resources, such as textbooks and course manuals, to provide familiar reference materials when reviewing details regarding diagnoses, assessments, and treatment methods. During your academic preparation, it is advisable to start a resource file box containing relevant articles and clippings regarding diagnoses and treatment ideas filed in easy-to-retrieve folders. It's never too late to start such a resource file.

Explore your fieldwork site's library. Many OT departments have their own libraries, or your fieldwork educator may keep a selection of references that he or she uses on a regular basis. Bring in your most applicable texts and share them with your supervisor. Frequently, these experienced therapists are excited to see new editions of their old reliable favorites and are interested in knowing about the kinds of materials you were exposed to in your academic preparation. Sharing your obvious interest in learning about a topic can lead to others recommending and even loaning you their preferred references.

Visit your local library and introduce yourself to the reference librarian. This can be a tremendous resource for treatment-related ideas. "How-to" books on subjects as varied as gardening, cooking, simplifying your work, time management, relaxation techniques, crafts, budgeting, and so on will give you invaluable ideas and instructions for developing fun and interesting occupation-centered treatments for your clients. You are likely to discover resources that will assist you in developing skills such as public speaking, teaching methods, and supervision that are required on the FWEF.

Visit web sites addressing specific diagnoses or topics for current information. They may have links to other helpful web sites as well. A list of helpful web sites is located in Appendix B of this book.

As you begin to treat clients, it is a challenge to remember details—sometimes, the remembered details regarding one client merge with those of another client. One method of storing information is to cluster or group such information. To accomplish this, try meeting and introducing yourself to the client before reading his or her folders, charts, or other documentation. Establish a mental image of the client along with a brief story about him or her. Then, when you read about this client or discuss him or her with other team members, you will be able to associate a face and a context with which to store the information.

Orient Yourself to Documentation

Collect samples, while protecting confidentiality, of documentation from the fieldwork site, selecting those that appear to be well written and easy to follow. Collect samples of notes written by your supervisor or other occupational therapy practitioners at the site, highlighting well-crafted phrases, justifications, and explanations. Many of these can serve as templates when developing your own collection of well-written notes.

Collect blank forms of each type of note used at the facility and fill in the type of information that is expected in each note or evaluation report. Study the site's forms, and find out where you can locate the resources to complete the information called for in the different sections of the documentation. For example, one section of the evaluation form may call for you to indicate the name of the wheelchair vendor available through the patient's HMO. Your fieldwork site may have a list of approved durable equipment vendors located in a card file on the front desk of the nursing station. You could then write this information in the corresponding blank on the sample evaluation form. Having done so, you will know where to look for this information when writing subsequent evaluations. Having a place to turn for such seemingly trivial information can save you numerous duplications of effort. Such preplanning can also reduce the number of instances you ask your supervisor for this information.

Develop a list of frequently misspelled words or unfamiliar vocabulary with definitions. Students have kept this list and the aforementioned documentation samples in plastic sleeves on clipboards along with their weekly schedules for convenient reference throughout their fieldwork day. If you perceive problems with spelling or use of proper terminology, it is advisable to also carry and use a simple, pocket-sized dictionary or electronic spell checker.

STRATEGIES FOR THE MIDDLE AND FINAL WEEKS OF FIELDWORK

Many of the strategies for meeting the fieldwork objectives for the initial weeks may be equally useful to implement or expand when addressing more advanced objectives. Review previous strategies and select those that seem applicable to your individual needs as you progress through the middle and final weeks of your fieldwork experience. In addition, consider the following suggestions that seem more appropriate as your basic skill level and confidence increase.

Network with other students affiliated with the same fieldwork site, or establish contacts with a few of your trusted friends from your OT academic program. Brainstorm some of your treatment ideas with these peers for feedback before implementing them. Acquire ideas for additional strategies for meeting the fieldwork objectives, and share some of yours. Though it may be tempting to share complaints about your fieldwork with peers, it is often counterproductive to meeting your fieldwork objectives. Try to stay focused on finding strategies and resources for success.

Arrange to observe your supervisor or another practitioner at the site while he or she is engaged in client treatment. Record in detail what they are doing—both the practitioner and the client. Later, review your observation notes, and provide a reason for why you think they are doing what they are doing. Next, reflect upon those assigned clients who could benefit from similar treatment ideas, and outline an argument for the pros and cons of using such ideas for the particular client. Share your observations and ideas with your supervisor for feedback. You will probably gain valuable information regarding how a competent, proficient, or expert therapist uses his or her clinical reasoning skills, and you will probably be able to adjust or strengthen your reasoning skills accordingly.

Arrange to have one of your treatment sessions videotaped. Initially, students (including, at one time, one of the authors of this chapter) balk at such a threatening idea. If the client is amenable and you can muster the fortitude to endure it, this can be an invaluable learning tool. Generally, people report quickly, forgetting they are being taped, and resume their natural behaviors. Because it is for your benefit alone, the tape does not have to be shared with anyone. However, after studying the results, you may want to view it with your supervisor or a trusted mentor similarly skilled as your supervisor for critique and suggestions for improvement.

If problems should arise during your fieldwork, do not hesitate to contact your academic fieldwork coordinator or the academic advisor assigned to supervise you on fieldwork. It has been the experience of some academic fieldwork coordinators that students wait too long before seeking appropriate assistance. You can keep your conversation confidential and receive the advice you need to approach the problem. Be sure to review the site's student objectives and write down specific instances of behaviors that you think document your progress toward meeting those objectives. This will help while developing a plan for alleviating problems, and both you and your supervisor may become more aware of your strengths as well as areas for improvement.

GUIDED EXERCISES

The following exercises have been developed to aid the student in successfully meeting fieldwork objectives. The strategy used requires the student to engage in active and systematic decision making along with problem-solving skills to resolve a potential dilemma. Remember, there are often several correct options available to address a problem. These exercises are designed to help you understand how you make decisions and to consider alternatives. Think creatively as you work through these exercises.

Problem One

Julie, an OT student, has completed more than half of her fieldwork experience in an outpatient clinic. During her midterm feedback, her supervisor identified that Julie should complete more evaluations during the remainder of the fieldwork experience. Julie had only completed one client evaluation, with substantial assistance from her supervisor, at the midterm point of her fieldwork experience. The fieldwork objectives clearly state that she is expected to independently complete four assessments by the end of her fieldwork experience. She has now been asked to evaluate a client using an assessment instrument that she has never used nor seen administered. This assessment is not listed in the fieldwork objectives. The evaluation is scheduled for the next day. Julie is very concerned about this situation.

➠ Identify three distinctly different options Julie could exercise in this situation.

➠ How would you rank the appropriateness of the options you developed, and why did you rank the options in that order?

Ranking the options and providing a reason for the order of options will allow you to examine your potential bias in decision-making skills. Did you arrange your options according to the amount of energy expenditure needed to exercise this option? In other words, did you select the easiest option as your first option? Did you arrange your options according to the potential response from the supervisor? Was your decision based on fear? Are you unable to identify options and arrange them in order because you feel there is insufficient information? Are you unable to experiment in the decision-making process?

➠ What resources could Julie use to help her with this situation? Identify at least three resources that she could use to help her decide which option to select.

➠ What would be the possible consequencs of any of the three options you selected? Consider the implications of each option in the near future for Julie, as a student at this site.

Problem Two

Sam is an OTA student in the third week of his fieldwork experience at a small community-based outpatient center. His supervisor has asked him to instruct the family members of an assigned client in the use of a specific piece of adaptive equipment. Sam has never used this equipment with this client. He knows that one fieldwork objective requires the student to instruct a client and/or family member in the use of adaptive equipment. This objective relates to the item on the FWEF stating that the student should be able to clearly give instructions. Sam feels poorly prepared for meeting this request from his supervisor.

➠ Provide three suggestions for Sam to address his problem.

➠ Identify the learning resources Sam would need to be successful with each option.

➠ Identify the potential consequences of each option you suggested.

Problem Three

Karen is an OT student who just completed the first half of her fieldwork experience in a large teaching hospital. During her midterm feedback session with her clinical supervisor, Karen was informed that she was barely passing the fieldwork experience. Her clinical supervisor used the FWEF and the fieldwork objectives to evaluate Karen's performance. Several learning objectives that were to be demonstrated by the student during the first half of the fieldwork experience had not been achieved. Karen had not completed assigned client notes in a timely manner, did not return the medical records to the appropriate location, and had failed to demonstrate independence in developing treatment plans for assigned clients. She was also frequently late for client appointments. Karen responded that she felt overwhelmed by the fieldwork experience. She reported that she understood the need to be mindful of the client's schedule and start treatment sessions on time. She also indicated that she was now using a schedule book to improve her organizational skills. Karen explained that she did not fully understand how to write the client notes. She also was not sure of the policy regarding the use of the medical records. Karen acknowledged her difficulties with developing client treatment plans and reported that she felt unsure how to prioritize client goals.

The clinical supervisor warned Karen that students do fail fieldwork experiences. Several strategies were discussed between the clinical supervisor and Karen at the midterm evaluation session. These strategies were to address Karen's midterm deficiencies and identify the resources available to Karen to improve her skills.

➠ Identify three problems Karen demonstrates in being able to meet the fieldwork objectives.

➠ Identify three strategies Karen should have used earlier in the fieldwork experience to meet the student objectives.

➠ Identify three learning resources Karen should have used to develop a basic understanding of the fieldwork requirements.

SUMMARY

This chapter discussed the purpose of fieldwork learning objectives and provided a wide variety of strategies to help you meet those objectives. Guided exercises were provided to support your learning experience as you read this chapter. The relationship between the fieldwork objective and the FWEF was explicitly presented with examples to demonstrate how both support entry-level competence. The fieldwork experience continues to be a very important part of your total education as an occupational therapy practitioner. This chapter also discussed the importance of developing sound clinical reasoning skills, not only to successfully complete your fieldwork experience, but to also provide you with the foundation for entry-level skills as an occupational therapy practitioner.

REFERENCES

American Occupational Therapy Association. (1983). *Fieldwork evaluation form for the occupational therapy assistant student.* Rockville, MD: Author.

American Occupational Therapy Association. (1987). *Fieldwork evaluation form for the occupational therapist.* Rockville, MD: Author.

American Occupational Therapy Association. (1996). Statement: Purpose and value of occupational therapy fieldwork education. *Am J Occup Ther, 50,* 845.

Buchanan, H., Moore, R., & van Niekerk, L. (1998). The fieldwork case study: Writing for clinical reasoning. *Am J Occup Ther, 52,* 291-295.

Clark, F. (1993). Occupation embedded in a real life: Interweaving occupational science and occupational therapy, 1993 Eleanor Clark Slagle Lecture. *Am J Occup Ther, 47,* 1067-1078.

Cohn, E. S. (1989). Fieldwork education: Shaping a foundation for clinical reasoning. *Am J Occup Ther, 43,* 240-244.

Creighton, C., Dijkers, M., Bennett, N., & Brown, K. (1995). Reasoning and the art of therapy for spinal cord injury. *Am J Occup Ther, 49,* 311-317.

Crepeau, E. B. (1991). Achieving intersubjective understanding: Examples from an occupational therapy treatment session. *Am J Occup Ther, 45,* 1016-1025.

Fleming, M. H. (1991). The therapist with the three-track mind. *Am J Occup Ther, 45,* 1007-1014.

Folio, M. R., & Fewell, R. R. (2000). *Peabody developmental motor scales.* Austin, TX: Pro-ed Publishers.

Hasselkus, B. R., & Dickie, V. A. (1994). Doing occupational therapy: Dimensions of satisfaction and dissatisfaction. *Am J Occup Ther, 48,* 145-154.

Herzberg, G. L. (1994). The successful fieldwork student: Supervisor perceptions. *Am J Occup Ther, 48,* 817-823.

Kohlman-Thomas, L. (1992). *The Kohlman evaluation of living skills.* Rockville, MD: American Occupational Therapy Association.

Kramer, P., & Stern, K. (1995). Approaches to improving student performance on fieldwork. *Am J Occup Ther, 49,* 156-159.

Mattingly, C. (1991). The narrative nature of clinical reasoning. *Am J Occup Ther, 45,* 998-1005.

Neistadt, M. E. (1996). Teaching strategies for the development of clinical reasoning. *Am J Occup Ther, 50,* 676-684.

Pedretti, L. W., & Early, M. B. (2001). Treatment planning. In L. W. Pedretti & M. B. Early (Eds.), *Occupational therapy: Practice skills for physical dysfunction* (5th ed., pp. 46-57). St. Louis, MO: Mosby.

Sands, M. (1995). Readying occupational therapy assistant students for Level II fieldwork: Beyond academics to personal behaviors and attitudes. *Am J Occup Ther, 49,* 150-152.

Schwartz, K. B. (1984). An approach to supervision of students on fieldwork. *Am J Occup Ther, 38,* 393-397.

Schwartz, K. B. (1991). Clinical reasoning and new ideas on intelligence: Implications for teaching and learning. *Am J Occup Ther, 45,* 1033-1037.

Slater, D. Y., & Cohn, E. S. (1991). Staff development through analysis of practice. *Am J Occup Ther, 45,* 1038-1044.

Zimmerman, J. (1988). *Goals and objectives for developing normal movement patterns.* Rockville, MD: Aspen Publications.

Note: Santa Cruz Mental Health and Substance Abuse Services, Community Connections, Craig Hospital, Rancho Los Amigos National Rehabilitation Center, El Dorado Center, San Jose Family Shelter, and Visiting Nurse Alliance of Vermont/New Hampshire provided the authors with their unpublished fieldwork objectives. The authors are thankful to these excellent fieldwork sites for sharing their objectives.

Chapter 3

PROFESSIONAL BEHAVIORS

Nancy Lowenstein, MS, OTR, BCN
Linda Duncombe, EdD, OTR, FAOTA

"When in Rome do as the Romans do." (unknown)

Professional socialization is the process of becoming part of your professional group in thinking and feeling as well as in knowledge and skills. When you began college, you carefully observed what others were wearing, how they carried their books, etc., in order to conform to the norms of other college students. Not that you did not retain your individuality, but you were in the process of being socialized as a college student. You have been preparing for the move from student to professional since you entered your professional curriculum. You have acquired knowledge that forms the basis for your profession, you have practiced skills you hope to use as a professional, and you have learned vocabulary to help you communicate with your fellow professionals. In addition, while on fieldwork, you will need a similar awareness of the social mores of the group you will be joining.

The purpose of this chapter is to help you to understand professional behaviors and the part they play in the fieldwork portion of your role as a student occupational therapy practitioner. By the end of this chapter, you should learn the following:

➡ Professional behaviors.

➡ Evaluation of professional behaviors.

➡ Attitudes and values.

➡ Professional appearance/presentation.

➡ Boundaries.

➡ Communication.

➡ Initiative and flexibility.

➡ Ethics.

WHAT ARE PROFESSIONAL BEHAVIORS?

Each school provides a student with the tools, knowledge, and skills to perform on a fieldwork internship. The ability to put the knowledge and skills to use in a real-life/real-time setting involves adding judgment and attitude to the academic piece.

In 1995, some physical therapists at the University of Wisconsin–Madison identified generic abilities for their profession (May, Morgan, Lemke, Karst, & Stone, 1995). These were defined as characteristics or behaviors that are not explicitly part of the profession's core of knowledge and technical skills but are nevertheless required for success in this profession. One of the generic abilities identified was *professionalism*, which is defined as "the ability to exhibit appropriate professional conduct and to represent the profession effectively" (Davis, 1998, p. 141; May et al., 1995). Other generic abilities identified were commitment to learning, interpersonal skills, communication skills, effective use of time and resources, use of constructive feedback, problem solving, responsibility, and critical thinking. Although this document was created for physical therapists, it certainly applies to occupational therapy practitioners.

Professional behaviors are a combination of judgment and attitude that identifies you as a professional—not just someone who knows anatomy or how to give a particular assessment, but someone who looks and acts like a professional and someone who has a sense of confidence; takes appropriate responsibility and initiative; is punctual; and is respectful to other staff, patients/clients, and family members. Although you may have received feedback on your professional behaviors from faculty, peers, and level I supervisors, you will continue to refine your professional behaviors during your level II fieldwork experiences and beyond. You will also refine your interpersonal skills as you build confidence as a professional. If you have concerns about your professional behaviors, you should feel comfortable discussing your concerns with your faculty, academic fieldwork coordinator, or fieldwork educator. These individuals, who are responsible for evaluating your professional behaviors, will be happy to discuss them with you. This aspect of your experience is so important to your functioning as an occupational therapy practitioner that a student will not pass internships without exhibiting appropriate professional behaviors.

EVALUATION OF PROFESSIONAL BEHAVIORS

The American Occupational Therapy Association (AOTA) *Fieldwork Evaluation Form for Occupational Therapy Assistant Students* (AOTA, 1983) includes an entire category on professional behaviors. Included in this section are time management; punctuality; clinic maintenance; taking advantage of learning opportunities and resources; modifying behaviors based on feedback; respect for clients' rights for privacy, dignity, and confidentiality; handling personal and professional issues in a way that does not interfere with their primary responsibilities; and adhering to policies and procedures.

The AOTA *Fieldwork Evaluation for the Occupational Therapy Student* (AOTA, 1987) identifies three categories of behaviors that make up the overall evaluation of an occupational therapy student: *performance, judgment,* and *attitude.* The *Guide to Fieldwork Education* (Commission on Education, 1994) defines these three categories by aligning them with the major domains of learning. The performance scale refers to the psychomotor domain in which the student is learning or showing proficiency in the technical and skill aspect required to function as an occupational therapist. The judgment scale relates to the cognitive domain. Judgment involves using problem solving and clinical reasoning to apply theory to carry out the process of occupational therapy, such as selecting assessments that will yield information related to issues of concern to the patient and to the treatment team, knowing when to move the patient to a different level in treatment, ending a treatment session if a patient appears to be in distress, and asking for help when appropriate. The attitude scale is considered similar to the affective domain. This is the feeling/tone that one uses when interacting with patients, family members, or other staff. This scale is frequently linked to professional behaviors.

ATTITUDES AND VALUES

"An attitude is a disposition to respond positively or negatively toward an object, person, concept, or situation" (Kanney, 1993, p. 1085).

"Attitude is the paint brush of life; it colors everything you do" (Sign in an elementary school, Newton, MA).

Because an individual is a representative of his or her professional group, actions and attitudes of each professional, when directed toward patients, colleagues, or society at large, are assumed to reflect the core values of the profession. The values accepted as core values of occupational therapy are altruism, equality, freedom, justice, dignity, truth, and prudence (Kanney, 1993). Embedded in these are commitment, dedication, taking initiative and self-direction (with an appropriate balance between autonomy and societal membership), truthfulness, respect for self and others, interpersonal competence, discretion, and moderation of one's self-affairs, among others.

When there is a discrepancy between one's demeanor and what one is saying, it may result in a misinterpretation of what one is trying to communicate. This may be due to an alternative meaning suggested by one's physical stance, facial appearance, gestures, or tone of voice. When one wears a nametag bearing a professional title but does not wear the clothes or accessories or have the overall look of a professional, one may appear unprofessional to the onlooker.

The rest of this chapter includes helpful suggestions for starting off on the right foot on your fieldwork experiences and for helping you reflect the values of the profession of occupational therapy through your actions and attitudes.

PROFESSIONAL APPEARANCE/PRESENTATION

Making the First Phone Call

You will be given the name and phone number of the person you should contact in order to schedule an in-person or on-the-phone interview prior to the start of your level II internship or to schedule your first visit for a level I experience. First, try to pronounce the name. If there is a possibility that you might have difficulty saying the name correctly, ask your academic fieldwork coordinator if he or she knows the correct pronunciation. If the correct pronunciation is still in doubt, be prepared to spell the name or say it in different ways to reach the correct person. If you reach an answering machine and the name is pronounced on the machine or if you reach someone who gives you the correct pronunciation, make note of it so that you will say it correctly in the future. Many people take offense at the mispronunciation of their names. This is one small thing you can do to start out with respect

toward your fieldwork educator at your site. This practice will be helpful later when working with patients/clients who may have unusual names.

Students sometimes complain about having to play "telephone tag" with fieldwork supervisors. If you are calling to set up a level I fieldwork experience, you will have to be persistent in calling frequently and at different times of the day. For level II fieldwork, if you do not reach the fieldwork supervisor on your first attempt, leave a message with your name, phone number, who you are, the reason for your call, and specific times when you know you will be at that phone number. It is frequently difficult for fieldwork supervisors to reach students at their dorms/apartments because the hours the students are in their residences are often the evening hours when therapists are not working. Suggest that you would be happy to call the fieldwork supervisor back at a time that would be convenient for him or her. Do not expect that the fieldwork supervisor will call you back immediately. Remember that the fieldwork educator's first responsibility is to his or her patients/clients. If the clinician is very busy, your message may be at the bottom of the pile. Wait at least 2 weeks before calling again. Start your second message with, "I know you are busy, but I was wondering if it would be possible for you to call me to schedule an interview." Leave all the information you left previously. Always offer to call back at a good time for the person if they will leave that information on your answering machine. Repeat this one more time after another 2-week wait, and then consult with your academic fieldwork coordinator about an appropriate course of action. It may be that you are calling too early for that facility, or because you were given the name of the fieldwork supervisor, that person may have been reassigned, or it may be more appropriate to make your request for an interview in writing.

Interviews are not required for all fieldwork placements, but they are highly recommended. Make certain that you understand what your academic fieldwork coordinator expects you to do in reference to scheduling an interview.

Interviews

Regardless of the kind of interview, phone or in-person, make sure that you refer to your interviewer by his or her formal name and title (e.g., Mrs. White, Mr. Green, Ms. Scarlet).

Phone interview: If you are calling the therapist, call at the time you said you would call. If the therapist is calling you, make sure you are there when the phone rings. Try to make certain that you will not be interrupted during the interview. If your call waiting beeps, let it beep. Place yourself, if possible, in a room away from others whose voices might be heard in the background of the call. If you are interrupted during the call, excuse yourself, deal with the interruption as quickly as possible, and apologize for the delay in the interview when you return to the call. Have something to write on to make note of information you will need for your internship.

Interview in person: Ask in advance if your interviewer would like you to bring anything with you, like health forms, your personal data form, level I evaluation forms, professional behavior forms, etc. Plan to take a small notebook to take notes if your supervisor makes suggestions of ways to prepare beforehand for the internship, such as specific assessments to learn, notes to review. Make sure that you are on time for the interview. Check the directions beforehand, look at maps, estimate the time it should take, and allow for additional time for getting lost or being held up in traffic. This may seem obsessive, but when I have a really important appointment to prepare for, I do a "dry run." That is, I go in advance just to make sure I know where I am going. If you choose to do this, realize that if you are driving on the weekend, the traffic patterns may be very different from the time of day you will be going for the interview. If taking public transportation, note any differences in the schedule from the day you do your trial run to the day of your interview. Make sure you know where in the building you will be meeting your supervisor and where you should park, if you are driving.

Dress

No jeans, sweatshirts, t-shirts, tennis shoes, hiking boots, or otherwise casual clothes. A nice pair of slacks and a nice shirt (blouse) or sweater would be fine. Do not feel you need to wear a suit, but if you have a blazer, that would be okay. Do not wear excessive make-up or jewelry. (I once had a student denied an internship because she was wearing too much "gold." The clinicians at the facility felt that she would not be able to empathize with their very poor clientele.) Your clothes should fit you well, but not be tight-fitting. You will need to move around, sometimes on mats with patients, and your interviewer may want to see what you think is appropriate dress. Also, tight-fitting clothing is unacceptable in mental health facilities, in schools, or in community settings where there may be a problem with boundaries. Hair should be clean, tidy, and off the face. During your initial phone call, it would be wise to ask about dress code if you have an unusual hairstyle, visible body piercing, or tattoos. Be prepared. You might be asked to modify your appearance based on facility policies.

Content

Unless you can talk to a student who has recently had an interview with a particular supervisor at a specific facility, there is no way of knowing the exact content of the interview. Some supervisors just like to meet the student, show the student the facilities, and tell the student about what will be expected while on the internship. The other end of the spectrum is the fieldwork educator who has specific questions to ask you and will determine from your responses if you will be accepted on the internship. In the event you might be asked questions of substance, you should prepare for the interview. Go over your notes from classes that covered diagnoses or populations you might be seeing at this facility. Rehearse your definition of occupational therapy. Practice "thinking on your feet" (e.g., if your supervisor asks what you will do if you are working with a patient bedside and you notice a change in the patient's respiration, what will you say?).

You may ask questions, too. You should prepare for the interview by looking over all the material available from your fieldwork office at your school. There should be a fieldwork data form that indicates the size of the facility, the ages of the people seen, routine diagnoses, types of assessment, treatment provided, etc. Included here is a form for you to use to help you identify questions for your interview (see *Questions to Ask During Your Interview* on p. 27).

Thank-You Notes

Almost immediately upon completion of the interview, you should write a thank-you note. The thank-you note can be on nice stationery or a note card, but unless your supervisor told you to call him or her by his or her first name, you should address it to Mr. (last name) or Ms. (last name). Keep in mind that this is different from the formal letter you will write to accompany your personal data form. That letter should be in business format. E-mail thank-you notes or electronic cards are not acceptable.

Apologies/Accepting Guilt

If at any point there is a misunderstanding about times to return calls, where to meet for an interview, etc., it is almost always in your best interest to accept the blame. Saying, "I'm very sorry; I must have misunderstood" will give you more stature in the eyes of your supervisor than if you go back and forth about

QUESTIONS TO ASK DURING YOUR INTERVIEW

	From the Fieldwork Data Form	*Questions to Ask*
Working hours— evenings? weekends? holidays?		
Dress— name badge required? lab coat? school patch?		
Transportation— public transportation? parking?		
Directions to get to the department from the lot or front door?		
Meals— Are meals provided? Is there a place to buy lunch? Do people bring lunch?		
If there is housing— When can I arrive? Where do I go to get a key?		
When are health forms required?		
If a criminal background check is required, is there a hospital procedure to follow?		
Prior to coming should I be— competent in assessments? if so, which ones? up-to-date on specific treatment techniques/diagnoses?		

the communication only to find out that you were right. Although you might feel better about this, think about what damage it might do to your relationship with your supervisor. Consider the slim possibility that it actually might have been your fault. Admitting guilt right away moves the conversation on to more important topics, and your supervisor may not even remember the incident later. Instead, you will come across as being a responsible person who is willing to admit when he or she is wrong.

BOUNDARIES

It is important to remember at all times that you are a student. You are a guest in the facility in which you have been accepted as a level I or level II intern. Act as you would when you are a guest in someone's home— offer to help whenever you see something that you think could be tended to, say "please" and "thank you," ask before you use something that belongs to someone else (this includes the telephone), ask if what you are doing bothers someone in your immediate vicinity if you are making noise, if you use something, put it away, etc. (I know this may sound like mother talking, but it is not my advice. It came from a student who was sharing her experiences with students who were about to go out on their internships. I have forgotten her name, but her brilliance will long be remembered.)

There are many benefits to the student role. You are learning and have the right to not know everything or do everything correctly. Once you have your license, you will never again have this special classification. Remember, you are practicing under the license of your supervisor. For this reason, you need to make sure that your supervisor can trust that you will do and say the right things at the right time. If your supervisor is not comfortable with what you are doing and wants you to practice a particular skill more before using it on a patient alone, you have to respect his or her judgment.

It is your responsibility to know the policies and procedures of the facility. If something was not covered in the orientation that you need to know, ask. In the same vein, be clear on the expectations that your supervisor has for you. Many students say that they did not know they were expected to do research about a patient's diagnosis or read past notes to get an idea of how they are written in that facility and wonder why they have been reprimanded for writing letters to friends, reading a book, or calling someone on the phone when they were not scheduled to be doing something specific. The entire time that you are in the facility, you should be productive. You are acting "as if" you are a full-fledged therapist and need to get as much as you can out of this experience.

Personal Concerns

You are human and will, from time to time, have something personal to deal with during the time that you are on your internship. You are expected to take care of those issues so that they do not interfere with the performance of your duties. Also, you should not burden others with what is going on in your personal life. If you need to make a personal phone call during the day, such as to make a dentist appointment, try to do it on your lunch break. If there is a reason that this is impossible, look for a convenient time in your schedule, and then clear with your supervisor that this is a good time for you to make an important phone call.

Although you may have a cell phone and need to have it with you while you are commuting, you should turn it off during working hours. This is especially important in a hospital setting where the electronics of a cell phone may interfere with life-saving equipment. In this case, the cell phone must be turned off before entering the building. In addition to the fact that cell phones may not be allowed in hospitals, the ringing of a personal cell phone is inappropriate in any setting in which you are concentrating on your professional role.

If you are upset about something, like an argument with a friend or family member, do not talk about it with your patients while you are treating them. The focus during treatment is on the patient. This is not to say that you cannot "chit-chat" about mundane things during a patient's treatment session, if it does not distract the patient and it helps the patient feel more comfortable, but just as you will keep information about the patient confidential, keep your own information confidential. Never agree to meet a patient outside of the hospital setting or after you have completed your internship and never give a patient your address or telephone number.

Maintenance of Physical Environment

Most facilities have staff who are responsible for cleaning, but there is no one who will straighten up or put away therapy items that you have gotten out to use with a patient. In addition, if you are working in a large department, there may be a rotation of responsibilities for cleaning up a splinting area, kitchen, etc. You should take your turn like all staff members, but it will be much appreciated if you pick up items that you see lying around, even if you were not the one to use them.

Responsibility/Dependability

It is very important that you arrive on time. This does not mean that you should arrive at 8 AM if you have a patient scheduled at 8 AM, even if that is the time your workday is scheduled to begin. You should arrive ready to work at 8 AM. If the time it takes to get to your internship is unpredictable because of traffic or public transportation, plan to arrive early. Then you can relax and get yourself organized for the day. It is better to err on the side of being early than to arrive late. If there is a major delay in your commute and you cannot avoid being late, call if you can to let your supervisor know. If this is impossible because you are on a bus in traffic, you will need to be prepared to apologize when you arrive. Most will be sympathetic to this happening once or twice during an internship, but not more than that. If there is a routine problem, you will need to problem solve how to change the situation so that this does not continue.

Sick days, vacations, and holidays are always a big topic of conversation among my students. **Level II students are not entitled to any sick days.** Facilities may grant up to 1 sick day a month if a student is actually sick. More sick days will result in your having to add time to the end of your level II internship. Do not ask if you can take a day off because you have not used your sick day. If you are sick, call your fieldwork educator as soon as you can to alert him or her to the fact that you are very ill and are unable to come in that day. Always offer to make up the time and the work.

Students frequently have family events to attend and need more than a weekend. If you are going to be in a wedding and need travel time to get there, it is best to ask about this during your initial interview or in your introductory letter sent 6 weeks before the beginning of your internship. Most people can arrange for times like this in advance, but remember that no one likes a surprise. Obviously, if there is a death in the family, you may have no advance notice, but whenever possible, ask as far in advance as you can. I always tell my students, "You can ask anything. What is important is how you ask and that you are prepared for the possibility that the answer might be no." So, how to ask: Always start your request with something like, "I know that I am not entitled to any days off during my internship, but I have been asked to be in my friend's wedding on [date], and I won't be able to make the rehearsal unless I leave by noon on Friday, [date]. Would it be possible for me to leave at noon on that date? I'd be happy to make up the time by staying late for several days or working some evening or weekend on a project for the department."

Holidays: Your supervisor will tell you what holidays you will not have to work during your internship. Schools typically have more holidays than most other facilities. Be aware that you may have to extend your internship by up to a week to make up for numerous holidays. Hospitals typically have the fewest holidays. Frequently, some staff work all holidays except for Thanksgiving Day or Christmas. It would be wise to not assume that you will have a particular holiday off. Several of my students have assumed that they would not have to work on Thanksgiving Day and the day after and have bought nonrefundable tickets to visit their families, only to be told that they were expected to be at work on the day after Thanksgiving. The moral of the story is to not make any plans without checking first with your supervisor about your schedule. If you need to be home to celebrate a religious holiday, address this concern with your supervisor in your interview or your introductory letter. Make sure you check the calendar in advance so that you can anticipate anything that might come up.

COMMUNICATION

Communication is the process by which humans share and interact with each other. We do it so much that we do not often think about how we sound, what we say, or what our nonverbal signs are. Yet, all these go into making up the complex interactions that are a part of communication. Many books have been written about communication, and it is strongly recommended that, if this has not been discussed in your curriculum, you read one of them or you review what you did learn about communication before any fieldwork experience. Communication is composed of both verbal and nonverbal aspects, and in the occupational therapy profession, written communication is important.

All communication involves a sender, a receiver, and a message. Additionally, part of the process involves feedback and the environment in which the interaction takes place. How did receivers actually hear what you said? Did they filter it from their point of view and only hear what they wanted to hear? What was the tone of voice that you used, what other nonverbal messages did you send, and what was the content of the message? Did you blame or accept responsibility? Did you explain clearly in layman's terms or did you use the professional jargon that you learned in school? How many times have you said something to someone that you thought was perfectly clear, only to have them misunderstand you? This is the dynamic of communication. When you are involved in a fieldwork setting, it is very important to try to be as clear as you can in your communication. How do you do this?

In your verbal communication, it is important to be engaged in active listening. One does this by both verbal and nonverbal means. By restating what the person has said or through clarifying and reflecting on the message received, you show the person that you are trying to understand his or her message. Additionally, through your nonverbal communication, you send a message of being engaged or disengaged in the interaction. You need to be aware of your nonverbal behavior when you speak with someone. Do you appear interested by nodding your head, leaning forward in your seat, etc., or do you appear nervous and fidgety? Do your legs

---

ACTIVE LISTENING

1. Think about a recent situation that took place in which you were not satisfied with the results. This could be with a roommate, coworker, friend, or teacher. Write down the specifics of the situation (i.e., dirty dishes always left in the sink; you always have to wash them; this makes you angry, etc.).

2. Next, write down what you remember you did or said. Include your tone of voice. Were you sitting or standing? How was your position in reference to the other person's? What were the other nonverbal signals you gave? What were those that you responded to from the other person?

3. Now, write down a new script. In this script, use "I" statements. Acknowledge the other person's situation, state the problem from your point of view, and suggest a solution. Think about possible responses that the other person might have, even role-play with a different person.

4. Now that you have thought through the communication barriers that originally took place, thought about a new way of approaching the issue, and role-played through it, try the real thing. Approach the individual, and try to communicate your concerns using your scripted version, remembering to keep "I" statements, reflect, and acknowledge the other person's feelings as well. I bet you work it out and feel better about the communication.

---

shake, or do you play with your hair, jewelry, or coins in your pocket? Try to be aware of your nonverbal signals. Start by asking good friends how they perceive these, and then try and become aware of them yourself (see *Active Listening*).

Verbal

What is the tone of voice that you use most frequently when speaking? Is it shrill, loud, or soft? Do you speak clearly or mumble? If you have an accent, how well do you make yourself understood? Additionally, how you pronounce words and approach people are all part of your communication style. Try to make note of your communication style. Ask others (friends are best) to honestly tell you about your communication style and how they perceive you. Use this knowledge when you interact in a clinical setting with clients and their families, supervisors, and other staff members. This knowledge will go a long way to help prevent communication disasters.

Empathy

Other aspects of communication involve how you show empathy to others. This is especially true with clients. If someone has just experienced a devastating event, such as a cerebrovascular accident, and he or she shares how depressed he or she feels, it is not appropriate to say things like, "Oh, this is just a phase of recovery" or "I know how you feel." These statements do not acknowledge the client's feelings and could be seen as condescending. To show empathy is not the same as sympathy. The latter can appear more

as pity, whereas the former serves to validate and acknowledge the sender's communication. It is far better to say something like, "It must be difficult to see the changes that have occurred" or "What you feel is normal, and you can feel free to express these feelings to me" (see *Statements that Express Empathy*).

Communication breakdowns occur for many reasons. Some of these may be a defensive posture on someone's part, a language or cultural barrier, or judgmental responses. As a health care professional, you need to be aware of your communication style, others' cultural influences and language skills, and your values and beliefs. A very effective way to avoid miscommunication is to use a technique called the *three-part response*. In this response, you first acknowledge/empathize with the receiver's situation. The second part is to state your feelings, and the third part is to suggest a solution. If you were feeling that you needed to discuss some issues with your supervisor, but did not want to wait until your regular meeting, using the three-part response, you might say, "I know how busy you are, but I am feeling a need to talk to you before our usual meeting. Is there a time we can talk today or tomorrow?" By using "I" statements instead of "you" statements and acknowledging the other individual's feelings or situation first, you have opened the door for good communication.

Cultural Sensitivity

Communication with those from other cultures requires knowledge and sensitivity to cultural differences. Learn about the cultural beliefs regarding nonverbal behaviors, such as eye contact, personal

STATEMENTS THAT EXPRESS EMPATHY

"Tell me more about that."
"How does that make you feel?"
"It seems hard for you to talk about this."
"You sound sad, upset, angry (insert correct emotion)."
"It sounds like you feel frustrated with your progress."

space, and touching. What are the beliefs regarding male and female roles and of disability in the culture? The best way to learn about another culture is to ask your client or a family member. Usually, they are pleased that you have asked and are willing to educate you.

You will be communicating with many individuals, from your supervisor to family members to other members of the health care team. Each interaction may require a different approach and different style of communication. Most problems can be solved with good communication, but will escalate with poor communication.

INITIATIVE AND FLEXIBILITY

As academic fieldwork coordinators, we are frequently told by clinical supervisors of both level I and II students that the traits of initiative and flexibility in students are the skills that mattered most to them. A student's academic performance did not matter because the knowledge could be taught, but the ability to be flexible and take initiative in today's work environment was essential to successful fieldwork, and these traits are not easily taught.

Taking initiative on fieldwork means not waiting for your supervisor to tell you what to do. It means using textbooks, journals, and new resources to look up diagnoses, medical terms, medications, and treatment ideas and not relying on others for their suggestions. It means keeping yourself busy if you have an empty block of time in your schedule by seeing if the clinic or work area needs to be cleaned up, observing another therapist doing a treatment, or making sure your paperwork is up-to-date. For many students, taking initiative can be difficult, as students often feel they do not know enough to take initiative and so they wait to be told to do something. As a student, you need to have confidence in yourself and to be motivated from inside yourself, not from others. It is preferable to ask

permission to clean up the clinic or research a treatment idea or diagnosis. If it is not okay, you will be told that. By letting your supervisor know you are thinking of these things, he or she will see that you are willing to do things without being told.

Flexibility is such an important trait in today's work place. Whether you are in a school, community, or institutional setting, events will happen that will require you to alter your schedule. Your client might be having a test done, be ill, or be on a field trip when you had planned to see him or her. Your supervisor may be out or may have forgotten you were coming that day (this happens for level I fieldwork more often than level II). If you are the type of person who has always liked to make a schedule and stick to it, then being flexible may be a problem for you on your internship or fieldwork. In life, things do not always go as we planned, and this occurs in fieldwork as well. You need to be prepared to change your plans based on your supervisor's, client's, or facility's needs and not to be angry about having to do this. Often, just knowing to expect schedules to change can help someone who is very organized cope with this issue.

Being flexible and having initiative both require good judgment and clinical reasoning abilities. Clinical reasoning skills are taught during your academic program, and you used them in different situations, perhaps in case studies or during level I fieldwork experiences. Clinical reasoning is a skill that you will develop throughout your career as an occupational therapy practitioner. As you complete level I fieldwork and then move on to level II fieldwork, you will feel that you do not have the knowledge base with which to make decisions. This is an uncomfortable feeling. However, with practice comes the ability to use knowledge gained from previous experiences. This is the development of clinical reasoning. It is important to realize that this is a process. Use your initiative to look up information, review previous client treatment plans, and make decisions based on this information. Using good judgment in this matter is key.

ETHICS

"The Occupational Therapy Code of Ethics is a set of principles that applies to occupational therapy personnel at all levels. These principles to which occupational therapists and occupational therapy assistants aspire are part of a lifelong effort to act in an ethical manner. The Guidelines to the Occupational Therapy Code of Ethics are overarching statements of morally correct action. The Guidelines also indicate a level of expected professional behavior. The Guidelines can be used to provide clarification when a perplexing problem arises, can be used as educational or supervisory tools, and can be used to educate the public" (Hanson, 1998).

As a student and an occupational therapy practitioner, you are expected to know and adhere to the profession's Code of Ethics. This document should be familiar to you from your academic program. Claiming to not know the Code of Ethics is an unacceptable excuse for ethical misconduct. Students often wonder what possible ethical dilemmas could happen to them on fieldwork. The answer is plenty. You may see a clinician billing incorrectly or not providing appropriate treatment, or you may be asked to provide a treatment that you believe you are not competent to provide. It is therefore essential that you be familiar with the AOTA Code of Ethics (revised 2000) and use this information appropriately.

Another important area is that of patient confidentiality. This is embodied in Principle 3 of the AOTA Code of Ethics (AOTA, 2000). You should never discuss a client with anyone outside the fieldwork setting using names or other identifying data. You may wish to discuss a client's case with faculty or in class settings, and this is okay as long as the individual cannot be identified. When one author was doing her fieldwork, her husband wanted to know how her day was, what patients she saw, and what their diagnoses or problems were. She had to quickly educate him that she could not tell him specifics about any of her clients. You may also need to educate your family, roommates, and friends about maintaining confidentiality. Additionally, discussing a client in the facility with people who are not involved in the case also violates an individual's confidentiality. Only share information with those who are involved with the client's care. If you are walking down the hall with your supervisor and want to process the treatment that you just performed or saw him or her perform, wait until you get to a private place to process this. Elevators in most facilities often have signs reminding staff not to discuss patients in this environment; the same goes for discussing clients at the lunch table with other staff. Be aware of who is around you and where you are standing when you discuss patients. Another area to be cautious is around telephones. Often, these are out in the open at nursing stations or in open offices. Do not take a phone call about a patient in one of these open areas. If necessary, ask for a phone number to call back, and go to a phone in a private area.

SUMMARY

The goal of this chapter was to give you some specific ideas and skills that pertain to professional behaviors while setting up fieldwork and when you are at a facility. Some of this may have seemed like common sense and it is, but to paraphrase a sign I once saw, "Professional behaviors are common sense, but common sense is not so common." How you present yourself in clinical settings is not only a reflection on who you are, but also on your academic program. With clinical settings requiring much from their clinicians, it is important that you represent your academic program well. Your attitude, appearance, communication skills, initiative, flexibility, and ethical behaviors are as important as your knowledge of occupational therapy theories and techniques.

REFERENCES

American Occupational Therapy Association. (1983). *Fieldwork evaluation form for occupational therapy assistant students.* Bethesda, MD: Author.

American Occupational Therapy Association. (1987). *Fieldwork evaluation for the occupational therapy student.* Bethesda, MD: Author.

American Occupational Therapy Association. (2000). *Occupational therapy code of ethics.* Bethesda, MD: Author.

Commission on Education. (1994). *Guide to fieldwork education.* Bethesda, MD: American Occupational Therapy Association.

Davis, C. (1998). *Patient practitioner interaction: An experiential manual for developing the art of health care* (3rd ed.). Thorofare, NJ: SLACK Incorporated.

Hanson, R. (1998). Guidelines to the occupational therapy code of ethics. *Am J Occup Ther, 52,* 881-884.

Kanney, E. (1993). Core values and attitudes of occupational therapy practice. *Am J Occup Ther, 47,* 1085-1086.

May, W., Morgan, B., Lemke, J., Karst, G., & Stone, H. (1995). Model for ability-based assessment in physical therapy. *Journal of Physical Therapy Education, 9*(1), 3-6.

Section II

FINDING THE RIGHT MATCH

Chapter 4

LEARNING STYLES

Beth O'Sullivan, MPH, OTR

One of the most critical components of one's occupational therapy education is the fieldwork experience, a dynamic program tailored to the individual wishing to attain the status of a competent entry-level practitioner. The Accreditation Council of Occupational Therapy Education (ACOTE) continues to place a very high value on this type of educational experience by continuing to support and to require field experience training in occupational therapy. This training must meet the ever-changing demands that occupational therapy practitioners face in everyday practice. To accomplish this goal, ACOTE has established a guideline for fieldwork training that includes experiences in a variety of settings that address all ages, disabilities, and various emerging practices within the profession (ACOTE, 1998a, 1998b). ACOTE also recognizes various levels of intensity in the training by mandating fieldwork level I and fieldwork level II. Both experiences allow students to continue their clinical education along a continuum, which will gradually increase the demands on the learners and will eventually lead them to their goal of becoming competent practicing practitioners.

One way of preparing yourself for this experience is to know yourself and your learning style. Learning and the style we use to gather information tend to be skills that we take for granted, not giving time or effort analyzing our own particular processes. It can be as simple as listening to directions or as complex as integrating a new theory of practice and applying that knowledge to individual clients. With deeper investigation of your own learning style and the process of learning as it occurs, you will be able to identify your individual style, and you will also be able to share that knowledge with supervisors in both the preclinical and clinical settings. It is also possible to acquire techniques through study under guidance that will expand your repertoire of tools that can be applied in your fieldwork training.

By the end of this chapter, you will understand the following:

- Learning style theory and the different learning styles or types.
- How learning styles are directly involved in fieldwork.
- How to address learning style differences during the fieldwork process.

Each and every person is a unique individual and will use different techniques to gather information and create meaning for him- or herself. Within this chapter, typical learning processes and several learning measures and theories behind these tools will be discussed. In reviewing these theories, you may be able to find several characteristics that are very similar to your style. You may also have had the opportunity to use some of these evaluative tools within your own academic background and have already discovered elements of your learning style. We will also discuss informal and formal ways to assess your style and how to operate within it in fieldwork experiences.

LEARNING THEORY

Several key factors are involved in the learning process and are described in a variety of theories throughout a review of the literature. Learning theories do differ in specific perspectives and in varying studies, but the process of learning tends to remain a constant within the literature. Many theorists have looked at the learning process globally and then identified specific characteristics that create an individual learning style, but how do we define style? Style can have several characteristics. The skill of learning can be broken down into categories, one being how we attain or perceive knowledge and the other being how we conceptualize the formation of ideas to then be acted upon (Guild & Garger, 1998). An example of application of learning on fieldwork would include how one obtains information directly about a client and then applies theoretical application and therapeutic concepts and formulates an intervention plan that can be implemented.

Perception is the initial stage of learning that involves the reception of concepts and ideas. It is basically receiving information. When some individuals perceive information, they may see the information for exactly what it is, while others immediately elaborate on the information and can expand it into different possibilities. Individuals may see concepts as a whole or formulate and compartmentalize ideas into separate entities. Some can attain knowledge from an abstract format such as reviewing texts and other resources, while others need to validate their knowledge through a concrete experience, such as hands-on demonstration (Guild & Garger, 1998).

Once information is perceived, it must also be processed in order to acquire and use the knowledge. Processing information is basically how one thinks. Some people enjoy taking information and immediately expanding on it in attempts to tie concepts together. A single thought or idea can be expanded upon and take an individual into a variety of new directions. Some individuals need to form an order to the ideas or information, and others are capable of putting information into groupings. Many people also use a variety of techniques to assist with the processing of information, such as talking out loud or repeating information verbally to gain a better understanding of what has been taught. Individuals may also act immediately on the information that has been provided, while others need time to process and reflect on the facts at hand. Think about yourself. Are you a person who tends to jump right in, or do you need to analyze the whole situation? If you are the type of person who enjoys jumping right in, you may want an affilia-tion that has lots of challenges and requires you to make quick judgments or quick change approaches to your client's care. On the other hand, if you need time to process information, you may want an affiliation that has a steady pace with several challenges and slower cognitive shift requirements.

Another critical element to learning is one's motivation or drive for new learning. Some people are internally motivated, while others require external encouragement and feedback. Those who seek feedback from others enjoy the outside opinion, while others are at least threatened or even see themselves as failures should their work be scrutinized by outsiders. This motivation or drive for learning may come into conflict if the supervisor expects a student to be motivated by being involved in the fieldwork process and have supervisors with experiential knowledge, when the student wants to complete the experience with high scores on the fieldwork evaluation form.

Environment also plays a critical role in one's drive to learn. Some people thrive in a fast-paced, competitive environment, whereas others need a quiet, low-key nurturing ground that supports the decision-making process. This could easily describe fieldwork sites as well. Some environments are highly competitive and require quick reactions to challenges, whereas others tend to be on a lower key with a more nurturing approach to one's individual speed of learning.

Newly learned ideas, facts, or behaviors must be acted upon in order to fully grasp what has been learned. Again, differences occur among individuals. Some like to analyze a problem and look at all aspects prior to moving ahead, while others will just forge ahead and immediately try to solve or tackle any part of the problem. Individuals may need structure to work and act within an environment with deadlines and time limits, while others may respond to a type of open-ended work situation in which jobs are set without a specified time or date of completion. Individuals may notice that they are more productive within a group, while others would rather tackle a task alone and remain in full control of a total project from beginning to end.

LEARNING STYLE INVENTORIES

Currently, there are many learning style analyses available for all students from elementary school through adulthood. Several tools will be discussed and have been identified as common instruments mentioned in the literature. However, those identified here are not meant to comprise an exhaustive list, simply a sampling. You may have been introduced to any one of the following studies as you have completed a variety of academic courses.

The Myers-Briggs Type Indicator was introduced in 1943 and was revised in 1976. It is a classic tool used to apply Carl Jung's theory in counseling to better understand certain personality and learning types as applied to education and business. Jung's theory basically states that people will perceive the world in two ways, either through sensing or intuition. Jung's theory has also stated that people make decisions or judgments by either thinking or feeling. This tool asks individuals to rate themselves on four very opposite scales. The scales are titled extroversion versus introversion, sensing versus intuition, thinking versus feeling, and judging versus perception. Through the use of specifically forced questions and word pairs, people are asked to make a decision that best suits them as an individual and will arrive at a measurement of where individuals lie on the scales as stated above (Claxton & Murrell, 1987).

Researchers Rita and Kenneth Dunn developed an instrument called the Learning Styles Inventory (LSI), which can be used in grades 3 to 12. Their Productivity Environmental Preference Survey (PEPS) can be used by adults. Individuals are asked a variety of questions and must rate them on a Leikert Scale ranging from strongly disagree to strongly agree. Through this tool, students are able to identify their own individual strengths in learning. Some of the areas evaluated are environmental, emotional, sociological, and physical. Subcategories are then identified to critically analyze each individual preference. Environmental stimuli include elements such as sound, light, temperature, and design. Emotional factors include motivation, persistence, responsibility, and structure. Sociological factors are identified in areas of peers, self, pair, team, adult, and varied. Physical factors include perceptual, intake, time, and mobility. With careful analysis of each individual's preference, one can adapt one's learning environment and work habits to meet individual needs (Guild & Garger, 1998).

David Kolb, another researcher, developed a specific theory and tool to assess learning style, coined Experiential Learning Theory. Kolb stated that learning is a four-step process. Learners tend to have an immediate experience that can be seen as being a concrete experience. Once they have become involved in that manner, they are able to reflect on it and gain different individual perspectives. From this process of reflecting on what is observed, people can form abstract concepts that can then form generalizations that will in turn integrate what has been observed (Claxton & Murrell, 1987). The learner will then use his or her own individual generalizations to guide and enrich any further actions. This form of active experimentation or actually testing what has been learned allows people to try their newfound skill in more complex situations. The continuous cycle allows people to compound original learning of a concrete experience at a much higher level. Kolb then categorized learners into four primary groups. The first are the *divergers* who grab onto the experience in a concrete manner and reflect on it using reflective observation. People who tend to fall into this category have the strength of being imaginative individuals and are great at brainstorming new ideas. This type of person is people oriented and can be quite emotional. On fieldwork, a student in this category may need to have all the information or scheduling in advance before feeling comfortable about scheduling a client on his or her own.

The next category Kolb identified is the *assimilators*. People in this group tend to gain knowledge through what Kolb states as abstract conceptualization and will manipulate thoughts and ideas to transform information through reflective observation. Individuals who fall in this category tend to assimilate very diverse information and integrate it into a whole. They love to create a theoretical model. A student in this category may become frustrated working within a health care system and dealing with outside constraints placed on him or her by the managed care environment.

The next category identifies people as *convergers*. Individuals who fall into this grouping tend to grasp the experience through abstract concepts and then must quickly use the information for themselves through active experimentation. An individual who uses this type of learning process leaps on a task and gets the job done quickly to reach the answer. A student in this category just wants to get the job done and may need reminding that he or she is one person who makes up an intervention team. The student may need to clear ideas or thoughts with the team prior to individual implementation of plans.

The final group identified by Kolb is the *accommodators*. These individuals grasp the experience concretely and transform it through active experimentation. Individuals who like this style focus on doing the task and having new experiences. Sometimes, accommodators have been risk takers and are so named because they can be seen as easily fitting into new situations (Guild & Garger, 1998). A student in this learning category may in some ways be a challenge to a fieldwork supervisor if he or she does not respond to the regimented guidelines and requirements or assignments placed on him or her at the site. This type of learner would benefit from encouragement to problem solve, develop his or her own individual learning goals, and develop personalized assignments to reach the identified goals.

An example of how you could incorporate learning style theory and teach to different styles can be found in the following assignment:

➡ Concrete Processing—Interview an occupational therapist currently in an area of practice.

➡ Reflective Observation—Discuss your thoughts on theories and the reasoning behind activities assigned by the supervisor.

➡ Abstract Conceptualization—Write a paper describing the site you visited, and address ways you could better serve the clients seen at this facility.

➡ Active Experimentation—Schedule another visit to the site, explore your ideas with the therapist, and actively implement some of your ideas with an identified client following approval by the acting supervisor. Reflect on the client's response to the intervention provided.

McCarthy developed a learning style analysis and teaching model based on Kolb's work. Through grant funding in 1979, McCarthy studied the four basic learning styles and added the identification of brain functioning and hemispheric specialization as applied to the individuals in each style. As a result of her study, she developed the 4MAT System (Guild & Garger, 1998), which identified learners in four new learning types above and beyond Kolb's original work. According to the new definitions, a *type one learner* will absorb information in a concrete sensing/feeling manner and will process the same by watching and reflecting. Someone who uses right hemispheric function will try to find personal meaning by completing the experience, but those dominated by left hemispheric function will try to understand the experience through the process of analysis. A person who is strongest in this learning style frequently asks "why" questions and attempts to integrate a personal meaning to what is to be learned (Guild & Garger, 1998).

Type two learners tend to perceive through the abstract and then process through the act of reflection. This learner uses stronger right hemispheric specialization to attempt integration of the experience at hand with what he or she already knows. A learner in this group who uses the left hemisphere predominantly seeks out new knowledge and asks the "what" question. Both right- and left-dominated type two learners tend to pay attention to detail and are precise in what they produce. They care about the validity of knowledge and respect the expertise of others (Guild & Garger, 1998).

Type three learners perceive information as abstract but must process information by experimentation to "prove what works." One with right hemispheric specialization will look for ways to individually apply the information, while one with left hemispheric specialization will attempt to answer any question by studying and observing what others have previously determined. People who function within this category generally want to practice and test the information provided by others in order to personally validate the facts (Guild & Garger, 1998).

Type four learners perceive information in a concrete sensing/feeling manner but will process the information by actively doing. These learners want to figure out all the possibilities and frequently ask the question "what if...?" The person who functions with strong right hemispheric specialization tries to explore possibilities or extend what has been learned, while the person who has left hemispheric specialization in this category tends to search for meaning behind what has been learned. Type four learners, either right- or left-dominated, attempt to see specific relationships between concepts, ideas, and facts. They enjoy watching others get excited about these relationships as they expand learning in general (Guild & Garger, 1998). It is the students' and fieldwork educators' responsibility to explore individual learning styles and expectations in the fieldwork setting and future areas of employment. Using the 4MAT system in both analysis of teaching and learning can assist an individual in adjusting to individual styles.

McCarthy's model also details that all teaching should address all learning styles (Guild & Garger, 1998). In doing so, the learners in each type find their comfortable area of learning and producing while also being exposed to other styles. They may even attempt to try and test other learning modes as well. Learners taught within this revolution of modes will profit because those who think in the abstract will be exposed to the concrete and those who deal best with the latter will be exposed to the abstract.

As one can see, there are many professional tools available to students. Even with this brief explanation of specific learning styles, you may have been able to identify styles to which you can relate or see aspects of yourself within those styles. Hopefully, you may have been able to complete a learning style inventory within your academic career. If not, you can certainly research any of these tools on your own and choose one that will provide more individual information about your own style. This may confirm what you have already determined about your style as you have analyzed your pattern used throughout your lifetime, consciously or unconsciously. You have instinctively used your style in many types of performance experiences.

EXPLORING ACTIVITY

1. How do you typically take notes when listening to lectures?
2. When writing a paper, do you have the radio on or do you need to be in a quiet environment?
3. In planning your assignments, do you give yourself extra time before the deadline or are you working up to the last minute?
4. When on the job, are you able to take spoken directions and remember them completely, or do you need written notes?
5. How do you organize your work and study areas?
6. Do you see yourself as looking at the whole picture, or are you able to analyze the parts of the whole?
7. How do you decipher the fundamentals within new theories or concepts when they are presented to you?

Knowledge of your own learning style can aid in future planning and fieldwork preparation. Realize that one's learning style can be adapted and changed to respond to a variety of environmental demands, even though you will continue to prefer established techniques or learning paths. Even if you have not completed a formal assessment, you may be able to quickly evaluate your preferred learning style. Some learning experts believe preferred learning styles can be divided into senses. In general, 30% to 40% of people are visual learners, 20% to 30% are auditory learners, 20% to 25% are tactile learners, and 20% to 25% are kinesthetic learners. You may even use two processing styles (Dunn & Griggs, 1998). A visual learner prefers to have visual demonstration and see directions. An auditory learner can pick up concepts and directions just by hearing them. A tactile learner prefers to use a hands-on learning approach, whereas a kinesthetic learner tends to use a combination of senses in order to learn, such as rewriting directions or notes and then highlighting them.

Look at how you try to gain information in various situations. *Exploring Activity* has several questions that can help you define your preferred learning mode.

Want to Know More...

If you are interested in further exploration of your learning style, you may want to complete exploration experiences in *OT Student Primer: A Guide to College Success* (Sladyk, 1997). A clear understanding of your style does not always mean smooth sailing on fieldwork. *Exploration Activity* (p. 42) provides some problem-solving techniques.

Becoming aware of your own learning style can be one way of preparing yourself for success in your affiliation. In researching your own style, a very important concept to consider when trying to make sure you can have success in your affiliation is preparation for the experience. Obviously, your academic experience is part of that preparation because it provides you with theory, concepts, and application techniques. Fieldwork is the time to apply and transfer your classroom knowledge to practical circumstances. Another means of ensuring success in the new experience will center around the interview process with your future fieldwork supervisor in the fieldwork site. In doing so, you will be able to articulate your background and knowledge of your own learning style. This will also allow you to gather information about the demands of the site and the expectations of the clinical supervisor. During the interview process, it is also important to explore the ways your supervisor practices and, if possible, determine his or her learning or teaching style. If you are a concrete thinker and your supervisor functions and thrives on extremely abstract concepts, you may want to discuss these differences. It is not important that you find supervisors who match your style completely, but it is important to have supervisors who can accommodate your style or help you develop other learning skills. Inherent in the fieldwork process will be your own continued expansion of your individual repertoire of style and improvement of application of theoretical concepts.

SUMMARY

Clearly, by students understanding their own individual learning styles and by having the ability to analyze future practice areas, they will be better prepared for future clinical situations and, ultimately, for employment. It is important to remember that we are all individuals and should respect our own and each other's differences in practice and learning. Matching

Exploration Activity

What can you do when your learning style is different from your fieldwork educator's style? Remember, you will always experience a variety of teaching styles and, at times, must adapt to the differences. Here are some techniques you can use to adapt your style to better match your fieldwork educator's style.

➤ Flex your thinking and try something new.
➤ Bring up the issue during supervision time.
➤ Practice the skill in your preferred learning style outside of fieldwork time.
➤ Try to approach some tasks in a similar way to your supervisor.

or mismatching of styles can be appropriate at times in order to expand the learning effect for all involved. Knowing one's strengths can be very helpful in assisting educators in understanding the areas of weakness to be addressed. Individuals, regardless of their similarities and differences, can be positive elements in any educational and clinical situation. The better we know ourselves and others, the better the total experience for all.

References

Accreditation Council for Occupational Therapy Education. (1998a). *Standards for an accredited educational program for the occupational therapist.* Bethesda, MD: Author.

Accreditation Council for Occupational Therapy Education. (1998b). *Standards for an accredited educational program for the occupational therapy assistant.* Bethesda, MD: Author.

Claxton, C., & Murrell, P. (1987). *Learning styles implications for improving educational practices.* ASHE-ERIC Higher Education Report No. 4. Washington, DC: Association for the Study of Higher Education.

Dunn, R., & Griggs, S. (1998). *Learning styles and the nursing profession.* New York, NY: National League of Nursing.

Guild, P., & Garger, S. (1998). *Marching to different drummers.* Alexandria, VA: Association for Supervision of Curriculum Development.

Sladyk, K. (1997). *OT student primer: A guide to college success.* Thorofare, NJ: SLACK Incorporated.

Chapter 5

KNOWING YOURSELF

Karen Sladyk, PhD, OTR, FAOTA

The concept of knowing yourself sounds like common sense. After all, who better to know yourself than you? As stated in other places in this book, however, common sense is not all that common. You likely know yourself as a student very well—you have had a lot of practice in that role. How well do you know yourself as an occupational therapy technician or professional?

This chapter is designed to help you take a serious and reflective look at yourself as an occupational therapy practitioner. The chapter will review your hopes, fears, skills, weak areas, culture, biases, and attitudes.

By the end of the chapter, you should be able to develop a proactive plan to avoid any possible trouble areas on fieldwork.

ULTIMATE GOAL

Other chapters have mentioned that every stakeholder in the fieldwork process has a goal. Although every student wants to learn and professionally grow during fieldwork, the student's ultimate goal is to pass. Failure to meet this goal means delayed graduation, increased costs, missing the National Board for Certification in Occupational Therapy (NBCOT) exam, not working as a practitioner as soon as possible, and, most seriously, the possibility of being forced to change your major out of occupational therapy. These are very serious consequences, so the better prepared you are to pass, the less likely you will meet these consequences.

HOPES AND FEARS

Let us first look at hopes and fears about fieldwork. Every student hopes for the perfect supervisor, someone who meets his or her learning needs in a supportive environment. Unfortunately, in today's workplace reality, that supervisor might not be available. There is likely less concern about level I fieldwork because, although you will feel nervous, level I fieldwork is typically very structured and has many supports in place. Level II fieldwork usually has bigger concerns because your professors are no longer there to help you problem solve, and you are likely to be in a one-to-one supervisory relationship with a fieldwork educator who is new to you. Take a minute, and review the list in *Student Fears* (p. 47). These are fears students report prior to level II fieldwork.

Stress has been well studied and is known to decrease cognitive functioning. When stressed, students do not perform at their highest level (Brown, 1999; Davis, 1998). The key to performing at your best is managing the stress that comes with the fieldwork experience. Of course, this is easier said than done. You already know that there are serious consequences to not passing fieldwork, including your school's policy on how many fieldworks can be failed before your degree is changed to another major. Stress is a natural part of learning. Why add additional stressful events to the fieldwork experience? Consider *Carlene's Story* (p. 47).

Students should work with their academic fieldwork coordinators (AFWCs) to identify possible events that might add additional stress to a fieldwork experience. These include a known or suspected disability, an unusual family situation, and life-changing events such as a wedding, pregnancy, or terminal illness. Often of greatest concern to an AFWC is how a student is addressing a disability, especially a mental health disability.

Students with disabilities are given the same accommodations on fieldwork as in the classroom, providing that the student self-discloses and the accommodations are reasonable. This requires a student to be insightful and open with the AFWC and the fieldwork educator. However, too many times, this does not happen because the student feels societal pressures to hide the disability.

When I worked as a clinician in a psychiatric hospital, I had a fieldwork student who refused to acknowledge she was anxious. I could see that she had all the symptoms of an anxiety disorder and that it was interfering with her functioning as a student. Finally, when I could no longer allow her to be with patients, she blurted out, "I have an anxiety disorder." I called the AFWC, who said she had spent months counseling the student to self-disclose, but she refused. I told the student that had she told me ahead of time, we could have avoided all the embarrassing situations in which she had put the both of us. If she were to be a good role model for all her clients, she needed to deal with her disability in a proactive way.

SKILLS AND WEAK AREAS

In the classroom, grade point average (GPA) is likely how you judge your worth in an academic manner. On fieldwork, GPA does not have any meaning. What matter are your skills. Students have been students for a long time, so their self-esteem is often tied to their GPAs. In the clinic, the fieldwork educator will want to see specific skills. In theory, GPA and skills should be strongly correlated, but often GPAs measure general concepts and not specific skills. A student planning for fieldwork would be more successful by assessing his or her specific skill level before choosing a fieldwork site. Use the questions in *Determining Skills and Weak Areas* (p. 48) to generate a list of skills and weak areas (see *My Skills and Weak Areas* on p. 48). Take this list of skills and weak areas with you when you meet with your AFWC.

CULTURE AND BIASES

Every time I mention culture in class, students groan, "We know, be respective of others' cultures." True, but culture and biases are more than respect (Wells & Black, 2000). Behaviors demonstrate your cognitive respect. When your culture is different from another's, your actions will show your understanding.

STUDENT FEARS

I'll be so stressed I'll...
Say something stupid
Freeze and not say anything
Blank out and forget everything
Forget something really important
Hurt someone
Not like my supervisor
Pass out at something traumatic
Throw up at something traumatic
Not "get it"
Look arrogant

I'll be so stressed out because I have...
No time
No money
Trouble with who I'm dating
Work problems
Family troubles
Car troubles
Other distractions

CARLENE'S STORY

Carlene was a senior occupational therapy student a few years older than her classmates. She had wanted to be an OT for a long time, but finances had slowed her progress a bit. She was a good student who worked hard in classes and was finally choosing her level II fieldwork sites. When meeting with her AFWC, she mentioned that she was engaged to marry her high school sweetheart who had been very supportive of her schooling. Because they were eager to marry and start a family, she would be getting married a few weeks after she finished fieldwork. The AFWC counseled Carlene that this was not a good idea because it would add more stress to the fieldwork experience. Carlene was confident she could manage it. She was good at managing stress and would plan ahead.

Her first fieldwork was fine, and she was pleased she was managing both the fieldwork and the wedding planning. Because she had planned ahead, a lot of the things she needed to do were already completed. Her second fieldwork was more challenging. Because the fieldwork educator knew that Carlene already had one fieldwork experience, she expected her to grasp concepts more quickly. At the same time, excitement over the upcoming wedding was increasing. There were surprise parties and friends asking to do extra things with Carlene. Carlene hated to say no; she wanted to enjoy the excitement of the prewedding plans, too. Her fieldwork caseload was increasing, and the clients were more complex now. She knew her number one priority was to be successful on fieldwork, but she felt gypped that she could not enjoy all this wedding excitement herself. Everyone else seemed disappointed she was not participating, too. Her parents were upset when she could not attend a neighborhood brunch, and her fiancée was saying she was "no fun, you only get married once."

By staying focused, Carlene was successful on the second fieldwork, but to stay focused, she missed out on the prewedding excitement that all brides should enjoy. In hindsight, putting the wedding off to a time she could have enjoyed would have been a logical plan.

Below are situations I have experienced with students. Consider what you would do with the following situations:

→ You are a male occupational therapy intern doing activities of daily living (ADLs) with a 70-year-old woman with a cerebrovascular accident (CVA). She cannot get her bra on.

→ You are a female occupational therapy intern doing ADLs with a 70-year-old man with a CVA. His underwear is all tangled.

→ Your 20-year-old traumatic brain injury (TBI) patient has photographs of naked girlfriends in his memory book.

→ The mother of your spinal cord injury (SCI) patient keeps putting him back to bed when you want to increase sitting tolerance. She says "it's her duty to care for him."

→ Your client has a day pass to attend a funeral and wake that you know will include heavy drinking.

DETERMINING SKILLS AND WEAK AREAS

➡ Considering OT content, in what areas am I most comfortable? Least?
➡ Considering OT theory, in what areas am I most comfortable? Least?
➡ When a teacher asks a question in class, how often do I have an answer?
➡ If a teacher stopped me in the hall and asked me to remember something taught last semester, could I recall it?
➡ When I separate my test grades from my project or other grades, do I see a difference?
➡ Am I more a long-term studier or a crisis-management studier?
➡ What do I know about my learning style that is an asset? What can get me in trouble?
➡ What feedback have I had in work or in school that I have not yet changed?
➡ How do friends and teachers describe me to other people?
➡ What positive attributes do I bring from outside OT to my practice?
➡ What would my entire faculty say about my skills and weak areas?

MY SKILLS AND WEAK AREAS

Name _____ Date _____

Skills	Weak Areas	Possible Plan for Weak Areas to be Discussed with My AFWC

CHOOSING FIELDWORK SITES

Good Reasons to Pick a Fieldwork Site
It's a "just right challenge," success is important.

Bad Reasons to Pick a Fieldwork Site
You want to work there after fieldwork.
You work there as a CNA/kitchen help and the OT offered to take you.
Your family member has an "in" there.
Your family member works there so you can share one car.
The site is close to home.
You are worried you will not get another spot.
The site is famous, and it will look great on your résumé.
They offer a stipend.

➡ Your client is HIV-positive because of a long history of drug use. He says he has never told his girlfriends of his HIV status.

➡ While working on mat activities, your client tells you that your religion is not the truth, and she prays for you to find the truth.

Be able to always ask yourself, is this a cultural issue that I only see my way? Is there another explanation to what I am seeing? How can I understand my client's culture to better facilitate occupation?

ATTITUDE AND A PROACTIVE PLAN

"Attitude is everything" say the hundreds of motivational posters you find in office supply and gift shops. If that's not enough, hundreds of self-help books in your neighborhood bookstore reinforce the idea. It's common sense, so why do we have to buy so many products that tell us this? Because human nature sometimes interferes. We sometimes do what we want to do instead of what we know is the right thing to do. Double-check your answers in My Skills and Weak Areas. How did you describe your attitude?

A proactive plan is a way to prevent problems on fieldwork. It begins with a positive attitude about fieldwork and your approach to learning. In Chapter 4, you assessed your learning style and what to do if your fieldwork educator's teaching style is different from your preferred learning style. Adaptability and flexibility is key. That same flexibility is important in developing your fieldwork sites.

You likely learned about the cognitive disability frame of reference by Allen. Allen advocates the "just

right challenge" for activities for clients with cognitive issues (Allen, Blue, & Earhart, 1998). After screening a client, the practitioner provides an activity just slightly above his or her current functioning. If the client is bedridden and dependent for all ADLs, you would not give him or her a wood trivet to complete. Common sense. The same concept is true for fieldwork; students should have a "just right challenge" considering their skills and weak areas. Too often, students choose fieldwork sites for the wrong reasons (see *Choosing Fieldwork Sites*).

As an AFWC, I arranged more than 1,000 fieldwork placements. For each "bad" reason above, I have several fieldwork "war stories." Consider the following:

➡ You want to work there after fieldwork: Fieldwork is for getting your feet wet, making errors, and learning. At the end of fieldwork, you will be a polished practitioner. Isn't that the better image to present to the place you want to work? If you struggled in any way on the fieldwork, you may not be offered a job ever.

➡ You work there as a CNA or kitchen help, and the OT offered to take you: The OT will not be the problem. The other staff who identify you as a CNA or other help are often resistive to seeing you in your new role. Students who have returned to their former job sites as fieldwork interns report that other CNAs often want the student to help with lifting or nursing asks for "extra pudding" from the kitchen. When reminded that you no longer have that role, staff are often offended you no longer want to help. Take a fieldwork site where you are you and not known for being someone else.

REDUCING FIELDWORK STRESS

Good Ways to Reduce Fieldwork Stress
Acknowledge it
Walk (or other movement) it off
Talk with peers
Set up a study plan with rewards
Call your AFWC
Set up a soothing home environment
Use positive self-talk
Practice relaxation exercises
Go in early and stay late to plan your day
Develop a schedule and stick to it

Bad Ways to Reduce Fieldwork Stress
Deny it
Plug through anyway
Blame others
Give yourself permission to not work to your potential

➡ Your family member has an "in" there: This has always been a mistake I strongly advise against. Once a board member who was a friend of a student's father opened a placement as a family favor. The OT openly stated that she did this only because she was "told from above." The student faced 12 weeks of knowing the fieldwork educator did not want the student in the first place. Take a fieldwork site where you are you and not someone with an "in."

➡ Your family member works there so you can share one car: In theory, not a bad idea but if one person works there, then often, the student becomes identified as "the son or daughter of..." Plus, any fieldwork problems spread like wildfire in the gossip of the facility. Once again, take a fieldwork site where you are you and not someone's adult child.

➡ It is close to home: Which makes more sense, a placement close to home saving 20 minutes per day commuting or a placement that offers a "just right challenge" that is further away? Even if you are traveling 1 hour extra per day for 8 to 12 weeks, you are only talking about 40 to 60 extra hours of your life for better success at passing the fieldwork experience. Use the extra drive time to be reflective of the experience.

➡ You are worried you will not get another spot: Talk to your AFWC about the reality of the situation.

➡ The site is famous; it will look great on your résumé: Famous fieldwork sites are exciting, but they often come with high expectations and demands. Make sure it is a "just right challenge"

and that you are willing to put in up to 40 extra hours in homework. Failing a famous fieldwork site does not look good on a résumé.

➡ They offer a stipend: Even if money is extremely short, do not pick a site just because they can help financially. Evaluate the obligations fully. Will you have to repay the stipend if the fieldwork ends? Are there additional hours required or expected? Are there fees or other expenses at this site that will negate the stipend?

Choosing the right site for you is the first step in reducing stress on fieldwork. During fieldwork, reducing stress can also be a proactive plan. Begin by looking at ways you cope with stress, as outlined in *Reducing Fieldwork Stress*.

I am reminded of a student who chose the coping skills on the "bad" list when fieldwork became overwhelming. She began by e-mailing faculty asking for lists of activities she could do with clients. When the faculty said that it was now time for her to look within and develop her own lists, the student told the fieldwork educator that the school had ill prepared her for level II. Next came e-mails that the fieldwork educator was "bad" and the site "inappropriate." After a site visit from the AFWC, things settled down for a few days but returned to the same self-defeating behaviors. The fieldwork was extended 2 weeks so that the student's stress level could be reduced and her thinking clear. In the end, she passed but wanted to write a letter of complaint to the site.

Using the coping skills on the "good" list would have reduced the above situation before it escalated out of control. Denial and blame not only increase the student's stress but require the fieldwork educator and AFWC to respond to the negative behavior. A proactive plan to deal with stress means a preemptive strike against the stress. Decide before fieldwork how you will manage a stressful situation. Involve other people in your plan of action.

SUMMARY

So now that you have read about all the things that might go wrong with fieldwork, you are likely feeling a bit stressed. No problem, it's better to learn from other people's errors than to experience them yourself. Remember, fieldwork is only 4 to 6 months. This is the only time in your career that you will be practicing under someone else's license, and you will be free to make errors under the watchful eye of your fieldwork educator. Your goal is to be judged by your future peers as a successful entry-level practitioner. Proactive plans begin with choosing the right site for your success, considering your strengths and weak areas discussed here. This topic is further discussed in the next chapter.

REFERENCES

Allen, C., Blue, T., & Earhart, C. (1998). *Understanding cognitive performance modes.* Ormond Beach, FL: Allen Conferences, Inc.

Brown, W. (1999). *Reaching your full potential.* Upper Saddle River, NJ: Prentice-Hall, Inc.

Davis, C. (1998). *Patient practitioner interaction: An experiential manual for developing the art of health care (3rd ed.).* Thorofare, NJ: SLACK Incorporated.

Wells, S., & Black, R. (2000). *Cultural competency for health professionals.* Bethesda, MD: American Occupational Therapy Association.

Chapter 6

CHOOSING THE RIGHT FIELDWORK SITES

Kathryn L. Splinter-Watkins, MOT, OTR

Choosing the "right" fieldwork sites can be fun and exciting, unpredictable, and anxiety producing all at the same time. Every student in an occupational therapy (OT) or occupational therapy assistant (OTA) program goes through a process of deciding which sites will best complete their education and prepare them for practice. Your original goals through this process can vary from finding the "closest site to home" to finding the "place for a potential job" to finding the "just right challenge" in a supportive learning environment. This chapter will discuss student concerns about finding the "perfect" fieldwork sites.

At the completion of this chapter, you should understand the following:

➡ What is involved in the assignment of sites.

➡ How best to work with the academic fieldwork coordinator (AFWC).

➡ Where to find information about sites.

➡ What to look for in choosing sites to best fit your particular needs.

➡ What is involved in accommodations to special needs.

➡ What happens when your fieldwork site is cancelled.

➡ What are possible optional learning experiences (different time frames, academic program requirements, specialty fieldwork/specialty knowledge).

➡ Whether to commute or live near the fieldwork setting: how to find housing.

The Selection Process

Occupational therapy and occupational therapy assistant programs vary in the ways in which students are able to select their sites for level II fieldwork experiences. This is because of variations in curricula, numbers of students enrolled, fieldwork site availability, regional and state differences, and individual fieldwork program methods at that college or university. Some programs require the students to find their own sites, some assign sites randomly, some use a lottery system to assign sites, and many programs attempt to match students to preferred sites. Chances are, the program you are involved in is a variation on any of the previous methods. It is to your advantage to learn how fieldwork sites are assigned at your particular college or university so that you can be prepared for that process.

The selection process that some fieldwork programs use is a lottery type of system in which your name is brought up randomly against a site name. There is little control over this process, and you need to be prepared to do your best no matter where you are sent. Some programs have you produce a list of possible sites or locations where you are willing to go, and you are randomly assigned to two or three from your list. Another process may entail putting your name into a hat or computer randomly for priority of selecting and then matching you to available sites as your name comes up. Some programs spend a great deal of time in attempting to match your needs with particular sites' programs and expectations. This works fine except that the unforeseen often happens to either the student or to the site, and it's back to "square one" in the process. Finding your own sites puts a great deal of responsibility on the student to ensure that you will not only obtain appropriate experiences, but also that the contract with the school goes through in a timely fashion for you to be able to go when you are scheduled.

Most schools have a list of potential sites with which they have contracts that are deemed by the AFWCs as valuable learning experiences that fit with their curricula. It is the responsibility of the AFWC to ensure that the fieldwork sites to which their students are sent maintain professional and ethical standards, maintain current contracts, understand their connection to the college or university and their role as fieldwork educator, and provide appropriate learning experiences for the students.

In other words, a lot of work goes into preparing sites to take students. Contracts or cooperative educational agreements between the college or university and the fieldwork sites must be completed. University or regional councils hold educational seminars and workshops, or coordinators give on-site fieldwork inservices to facilities in preparation for taking students. Many coordinators still regularly visit fieldwork sites (as budgets, time constraints, and teaching loads allow). At the least, new sites are usually visited by the coordinator before or while you are scheduled to be there. All programs, through phone contact and correspondence, both mail and e-mail, exchange information about the OT/OTA program curriculum and expectations about each fieldwork site, including administration, OT department, placement reservations, and planned fieldwork program.

Because this process of procuring and coordinating the availability of fieldwork sites takes a lot of time and effort, finding specific sites is not always a quick and easy task. You must realize that there are many OT and OTA programs searching for sites and sending students out at the same time that you will be going. Most sites take students from more than one school, take students only during a certain time of year, or take students only for a certain experience. Thus, not all sites are available at all times. Even if your coordinator accepts leads to potential sites, you should not count on having that site for yourself because of the time and different factors involved. But, it can be a possibility for students in the future.

Because of the constant fluctuations in the health care system and site or supervisor availability that are out of the control of your fieldwork coordinator, you should prepare yourself to essentially "go anywhere." The Accreditation Council for Occupational Therapy Education (ACOTE) Standards (1998) require that educational programs provide learning experiences that prepare you for entry-level competency. There is no requirement for specific types of sites or specific locations. It is up to your OT or OTA program to decide how it wants to meet the ACOTE Standards to prepare you for practice. So, if you are able to choose certain sites, practice areas, or locations, you must understand what is involved to make the best choices for yourself and your chosen profession.

At our school, we give a list of preferred sites from which the students choose. In preparation for selecting sites, I tell my students the following:

➡ All sites are good. All sites on the list are screened by the AFWC and should follow the same guidelines for practice and education.

➡ All sites are different. Each site varies by supervisor, staffing, practice area, philosophy of education, program structure, expectations, numbers of students, etc.

⇒ Each site is unique. Just as you are each unique and have different needs, so too are each of the sites and supervisors. As will be mentioned throughout this book, a positive attitude and flexible learning approach will make any site a successful experience.

Working with the AFWC

Although it may not always be possible to give you your "perfect" sites, things always work out for the best. One student writes, "Thanks for all your support. I was scared to death to go [to a newly assigned site], but I did, and I learned so much!"

The AFWC wears many hats: teacher, mentor, coordinator, manager, taskmaster, advisor, and supporter. As you choose sites, the one most familiar with different settings is the OT/OTA program's fieldwork coordinator. The AFWC will assist you in assessing your past experiences and educational needs, understanding the various types of sites and programs available, and coping with whatever happens along the way.

Three important words to remember when dealing with the AFWC are communication, consideration, and responsibility. *Communication* is fundamental for not only speaking up for your educational needs in a mature way, but also for getting all the required forms, corresponding with your site, and getting any special personal situations understood. Now, *everyone* has his or her own unique *desires* that may or may not be accommodated. What you want or desire may not be the same as what you need. The "special" personal situations referred to here include needs that are *out of the ordinary* that may truly affect your fieldwork performance, such as a disability, a hardship, or a particular desire for an extra learning challenge. Communication is also vital if problems arise at your fieldwork site. Your first contact for solving problems is your on-site supervisor and then the site's student program coordinator, if there is one. The main link in the chain of command—your advisor and teacher—is the AFWC, who will help you to problem solve through any situation with phone calls, e-mail, or visits.

Consideration is important, as the AFWC has many sites and students to coordinate, both on campus and on fieldwork, so be considerate of his or her time and of office space (if files are located there) and respect decisions made, as you probably will not know all of the parameters involved. The other area of consideration is for the fieldwork educators at the fieldwork sites. You represent your school. Be considerate of your site supervisor's time and efforts in providing an education for you. Being conscious of this helps to maintain that site for future students and protects the investment and site development efforts of the AFWC.

The third word of advice is to take *responsibility* for your own learning. If the available site is not what you had hoped, then take it upon yourself to seek out learning experiences through extra experiences at your assigned site, field trips to other sites, volunteer activities, part-time work experience, and workshops. The ultimate responsibility for your AFWC is to provide an opportunity for your education through fieldwork. However, it is ultimately up to you to develop your own life's direction and career.

Finding Site Information

The following are places to find information on sites:

⇒ Fieldwork data form

⇒ School fieldwork office files

⇒ Library

⇒ Internet

⇒ Student evaluation of fieldwork experience

⇒ Grapevine

Almost all AFWCs keep files or have files located in the library or on computer for students to peruse for information about sites. Whether or not you are able to look at the files before your site is assigned or after you have been given your assignments, you should know that there are a great many variations on practice areas.

The most reliable form of information is the Fieldwork Data Form (Commission On Education, 1999a). This is filled out by the facility or agency for the express purpose of giving information about its site to the student and the school. Usually, there are files located in the library, the fieldwork office, the OT/OTA department office, or on the computer. Files may also contain brochures, fieldwork objectives, possible assignments, housing information, and maps. The Internet is also helpful for obtaining general facility information and maps or directions. The student evaluation of fieldwork experience (Commission On Education, 1999b) is another resource, although you must take this with a "grain of salt," as it is only one student's perspective. As mentioned before, each student is unique in his or her own experience of a site. Two students may have the same supervisor, be on the same unit of a facility, and have totally different experiences and outcomes. However, it is a possible

---

RANGE OF EXPERIENCES

➡ Institutional to community agency to home based
➡ Inpatient facility to outpatient setting
➡ Acute care to rehabilitation to outpatient to home health
➡ Day care to preschool to specialty camps to public schools
➡ Traditional to innovative to potential OT sites
➡ Mental health to physical disabilities to wellness clinics
➡ Rural to suburban to urban settings
➡ Medical model to social model to educational model
➡ General to varied to specific service delivery
➡ Pediatric to adolescent to adult to geriatric to hospice

---

resource if it is available and may in fact give some good insight to a particular student's experience of that fieldwork program and may list possible housing.

The grapevine (or gossip) is the least reliable form of information, although it is usually what the students listen to first. Have you ever played the game where one person whispers something in a person's ear and the message is passed around the room? The last person repeats the message out loud, and it is totally garbled and misunderstood. This is how the grapevine works. It is baffling that one site can be the "best site ever" one year and the next year be shunned as a "place that fails everybody." Some crazy rumors get around. Do not believe everything you hear, and check for the facts with the files or with the AFWC. Know again that you are an entirely unique individual who will have your own experiences that are different from anyone else.

TYPES OF SITES

Practice environments range from institutional to community settings and from rural to suburban to urban or inner city (see *Range of Experiences*). Settings can vary from inpatient to outpatient clinics, from focused on a rehabilitation unit to traveling around for a home health agency, from a large university-affiliated medical center to a small community hospital, and from medically oriented to socially oriented. A setting can be specialized to work with persons with one specific diagnosis, such as Alzheimer's, amyotrophic lateral sclerosis (ALS), burns, hands, or traumatic brain injury (TBI), or it can be generalized to evaluate and treat whatever is referred, as in a general hospital, medical center, or rehabilitation facility. OT practitioners work with all ages, so it is recommended that the student get experience across the lifespan (ACOTE, 1998).

A new dimension in fieldwork is that, as our profession reaffirms its commitment to occupation-centered practice and education, sites can now be looked at as traditional (role-established) or innovative (role-emerging) (Bossers, Cook, Polatajko, & Laine, 1997; Dunbar, Simhoni, & Anderson, 2001). In the traditional or role-established setting, the OT practitioner has an established role in that work environment. Examples might include a medical center or school system where the student is expected to follow and learn from the OT practitioner's particular role, lead, and example. This is usually the most secure setting for a student because of the defined roles and structure.

In the nontraditional, innovative, or role-emerging setting, the role of the OT practitioner is not defined, and the OT program is not yet established. Students may have a non-OT supervisor and/or a part-time OT supervisor. Examples may include a homeless shelter, a community mental health agency, or a residential program for people with mental retardation/developmental disabilities where the student must work with non-OT personnel and create and establish the OT role. This is a great placement to challenge the fieldwork student to develop independent and self-directed learning (Herge & Milbourne, 1999).

Dunbar et al. (2001) add a third dimension of role-exploring in which the site would not have any OT programming and the student would have a non-OT supervisor and an off-site part-time OT supervisor or faculty. In this setting, the potential role of OT is explored and discussed with the off-site OT supervisor or mentor. Although not normally used for level II experiences, many universities and colleges use role-exploring placements, such as community day care agencies, community mental health day programs, and forensic settings, for level I fieldwork experiences.

In past years, the traditional fieldwork placements included one physical disabilities setting and one psychosocial disabilities setting, with the option of a third pediatrics or other specialty setting. Some schools required fieldwork in all three areas; others only required the physical and psychosocial combination. Now, even school systems, which used to be a specialty area, are seen as traditional or role-established. Choices are much broader, as ACOTE standards (1998) have evolved with practice and education. ACOTE recommends that the student be exposed to a variety of clients across the lifespan and to a variety of settings. The changing health care, legal, and reimbursement systems are driving the availability of placements from traditional and medical model sites to innovative and role-emerging practice areas. This puts a great deal of responsibility on the school and student to clarify and assert the role of OT in new settings.

In selecting sites for learning, the student must take into account his or her own attributes (learning style, attitude, readiness, comfort level) and look for balance and variety. For instance, pairing a traditional rehabilitation setting with a community mental health setting gives a broad spectrum of care continuum. Pairing a hospice home health setting and a children's medical center also gives a broad spectrum of OT practice in a more innovative combination.

Acute care or acute rehabilitation units (physical disabilities) are usually faster paced with lots of variety. This appeals to many students, whereas a nursing home (physical disabilities) that offers repetition of certain protocols and a few primary diagnoses, such as patients with orthopedic and neurological conditions, appeals to others. Although mental health issues should be dealt with in any environment, a fieldwork experience within a mental health facility or unit can be invaluable to one's understanding of interpersonal skills and therapeutic use of self. Many students look for fieldwork experiences with the pediatric population. Indeed, school systems are currently the biggest employer of OT practitioners (American Occupational Therapy Association [AOTA] Conference, 2001). But, there are many types of pediatric settings that will prepare you to work in the schools without actually having to do a fieldwork experience in the schools. Students share experiences in the following vignettes:

➡ Amy knew for sure that she was going to practice in a rehabilitation setting, but after she completed both of her fieldwork experiences, it was her psychosocial fieldwork experience that was most appreciated and led to her area of expertise with head injury clients. Unless you explore your values and push your boundaries, you won't know your talents and skills.

➡ Felicity writes, "Everything is going great at my fieldwork site. I absolutely love it! Working at this site has made me interested in working in a whole new setting (mental health)." Unless you try something new and go with a positive attitude, you will never discover the treasures and enjoyment in your life's work.

EDUCATIONAL NEEDS ASSESSMENT

The first step is to perform an educational/professional needs assessment (see *Fieldwork Experience Grid* on p. 58 and *Fieldwork Setting Grid* on p. 59). Look at experiences on level I, types of facilities, types of supervision, direction of own professional interests and goals, and any special personal needs. Within the grid, highlight the experiences that you have had at the various level I, volunteer, working, and classroom activities. The goal here is to obtain as well-rounded an education as possible.

There are other questions to ask as you look at completing and enhancing your education. In addition to level I experiences, what work or volunteer experiences have you had? What are your hobbies, skills, and interests? Where do you see yourself practicing in 5 years? What are you most comfortable with, least comfortable? Are you a concrete thinker, more abstract, or theoretical? To which practice areas would you like more in-depth exposure? In which areas do you think that you would like to work; which areas are not at all appealing to you; and which areas would help to round out your experiences in the OT world? You should end up with quite a variety of possibilities.

So, for example, if you have spent time in a community mental health center, pediatric day care, and nursing home during your level I experiences, you may need to look at doing at least one of your level II experiences in a hospital or rehabilitation setting for medical model or traditional OT/OTA role exposure. If, for instance, you really liked your mental health experience, you may want to experience this type of setting in more depth during a level II experience. Maybe you are really interested in working with children. There are several different types of settings that can give you experience with children, including community agencies, school systems, child psychiatric units, juvenile detention facilities, private practice, home health, developmental disabilities institutions, or specialty children's hospitals—all of these can give you exposure to working with children, but each is unique in how children's needs are served.

FIELDWORK EXPERIENCE GRID

List your fieldwork I experiences and any relevant work or volunteer experience:

Name of facility, city, state

_____

_____

_____

_____

Using a highlighter, categorize the areas of practice that you've experienced already as indicated above:

Lifespan Continuum	Disability Status	Environment	OT Role Continuum
Infant/child (0 to 2 years)	Well	Rural	Role-established (Traditional)
Young child (3 to 5 years)	Acute	Suburban	Role-emerging (Innovative)
Child (6 to 12 years)	Chronic	Urban	Role-exploring (Level I) (Potential)
Adolescent (13 to 18 years)	Terminal	Institution	
Young Adult (19 to 29 years)		Satellite or OP clinic	
Adult (30 to 65 years)		Community	
Older adult (66 to 75 years)		Home Based	
Elderly (75+ years)			

Discuss what areas interest you further and what areas you are missing.

FIELDWORK SETTING GRID

Using one highlighter, categorize the types of settings and/or service delivery you have already experienced. Using another highlighter, color in what types of additional settings and/or service delivery might give you a well-rounded education.

Setting/Service Delivery

Community Hospital	State Hospital	County Hospital	University Hospital
Large Medical Center	Government (VAMC) Facility	Specialty Facility	General Facility
Mental Health Facility	Rehabilitation Center	Community Agency	Private Practice
Psychiatric Unit (in hospital)	Rehabilitation Unit (within larger facility)	Subacute Unit	Neonatal Unit
Nursing Home	Hand Clinic	Outpatient Clinic	Forensic Site
Pre-School	Elementary School	High School	University Affiliated
Partial Hospital or Day Program	Community Re-Entry Program	Vocational Rehabilitation	Work Capacity Center
Burn Unit	Head Injury Unit	Spinal Cord Unit	Residential Facility
Not-for-profit Agency	For-profit Agency	Pediatric Unit	Adolescent Unit
Homeless Shelter	Hospice	Adult Unit	Geriatric Unit
Home-based (Home health)	Specialty Camp	Public Facility	Religion Affiliated

Now, step back and look at what experiences you have been exposed to and what experiences you might like to be involved with for your level II fieldwork experiences.

Adapted from EKU Fieldwork Selection Seminar, Smith & Splinter, 1992.

Remember that the level II experience is to prepare you for *entry-level general practice*. Also remember that you can always obtain additional experiences by volunteering or working (not as an OT or OTA) in areas in which you are interested. You should be able to problem solve from what you gain on your level I and II experiences, work, volunteer, and classroom activities to be successful on the National Board for Certification in Occupational Therapy (NBCOT) certification exam and wherever you go to work. You do not need to experience everything on fieldwork before you find your first job. A student shares her experience in the following vignette:

➡ Carmen stated that her first "job" after graduation was as a full-time volunteer at a summer camp for children with autism. This prepared her for her eventual job in the public school system when the opportunity became available in the fall. By taking advantage of learning experiences outside of school and work, you demonstrate your dedication and expand your marketability and skills.

SPECIAL NEEDS

If you have special needs out of the ordinary, such as an extenuating home situation, a condition that may need consideration during your fieldwork practice, or a disability that you have accommodated for through your educational process, it is important to bring up anything that could jeopardize your fieldwork performance with your AFWC. He or she will help you determine if it is something to clear or make accommodations for at your fieldwork site.

OPTIONAL FIELDWORK LEARNING EXPERIENCES

Some OT programs offer a third level II fieldwork experience. Doing a third specialty fieldwork experience is a great way to prepare you further for today's practice environment. Because you have been through two internships already, you would be starting out on a different level. A third experience offers a way to hone skills further or learn new skills in a new setting. Arrangements for this extra learning experience must be made through the AFWC and the school. Often, the time frame is variable (4 to 12 weeks), with the tuition varying accordingly. Although thinking about this before you leave campus is advisable, you can also decide to do specialty fieldwork while you are on your fieldwork experiences. The experience can be tailored to your desires for extra knowledge and practice because it is not a required part of the program. A student shares her experience in the following vignette:

➡ Jennifer writes about a nontraditional setting: "I have been extremely busy but am learning so much. Working with the members has been a great experience, and the staff members really have a wonderful appreciation for OT. I have decided to stay an extra 6 weeks for a specialty fieldwork."

One option to further prepare you for evolving areas of OT practice is to go the extra mile and stay for a specialty fieldwork experience.

If doing extra weeks of fieldwork is not possible, think about combining your required experiences in an innovative way. You may now combine one to four experiences within the timeframe required by ACOTE (1998). The minimum requirement for the OT student is 24 weeks of full-time level II fieldwork; for the OTA, it is 16 weeks of full-time fieldwork. Part-time (but not less than half-time) is also possible for a longer period of time. It is up to your school as to how to work this out. Keep in mind that the AFWC must still work out the contracts and coordinate the time and expectations at each site.

THE DREADED CANCELLATION

Cancellations work out for the best, believe me. When you are told that your next site has cancelled, it can be disappointing to say the least. However, you really do not want to go to a site that has to cancel. There are many reasons for cancellations, from staffing changes to program changes to administrative changes. Almost all of the changes are out of the control of you or your fieldwork coordinator, so this is when your coping skills and collaboration with your AFWC come into play. In almost every situation, the student has said, "I am so glad that I was able to go to this site instead of the one I was assigned to originally." It's amazing how things always work for the better.

So, what do you do when your AFWC calls you and tells you that your site has cancelled? This is a time for regrouping, reassessing your directions, and trusting in your AFWC to come up with something to meet your needs. Do not confuse things by searching on your own for sites. Unless your coordinator tells you that he or she needs for you to look for sites, you will have to rely on the fact that it is your coordinator's job to find you a replacement site.

If the cancellation is last minute (as often happens), it can be very difficult to find an appropriate replacement site, although every effort is made to keep you on schedule. Sometimes, the site will be further away or involve a different learning situation. If a site cannot be found in time, one option to consider includes sitting out for 2 months (OTA) or 3 months (OT) and going out in the next rotation. Although this is not something for which you can plan, sometimes this also works out for the best. (Take a well-deserved break.) With the NBCOT exam being given four times a year and soon on demand, the time between finishing and taking the exam is not as long as when it was given only twice a year. The main thing to remember is to stay calm and to assist your coordinator the best you can.

LOCATION, LOCATION, LOCATION

Many students request sites close to their homes. Although this is understandable, it is not always possible and not always the best for your education. Keep in mind that all faculty and OT practitioners have also done level II fieldwork. We have "been there and done that." All OT practitioners understand the constraints and concerns about family, children, spouses, pets, financial limits, and fear of the unknown. The primary purpose of the college or university that you are attending is to provide you with a good education, and the purpose of the OT program is to create a general, entry-level, competent practitioner. This means that part of that education may entail leaving home for 6 weeks to 6 months in order to do fieldwork at appropriate sites. As you look at the particular educational opportunities and the areas in which you are interested in practicing, you will notice that your best experiences may not be within 30 miles of home. Thus, to get the best education, you will have to problem solve where to live. Crist (1996) advises not to let the housing issue determine your fieldwork site. Some students decide to commute up to 2 hours a day to their site for fieldwork. This can be stressful in itself, as the days can be intense and the drive long and wearing, but the reward of an excellent site is worth the extra drive.

Many other alternatives are available to those who are creative. Below is a partial list of suggestions and resources:

➡ Check the AOTA web site (www.aota.org) under the Student Area. The "Level II Survival Guide" has many tips.

➡ Contact local universities and colleges for possible housing options.

➡ Call local senior citizen centers about seniors living independently in need of a companion. Often, you can trade errands, minor repairs, or companionship for room and board.

➡ Speak with local churches or community groups about connections with people they might know in the city to which you will be going.

➡ Review potential contacts in areas where you will be going, such as family or extended family, family friends, or a classmate's family.

➡ Check out the Chamber of Commerce for leads on housing and community resources.

➡ Check out the classified advertising sections in the local newspapers.

➡ Check out the Internet for leads on housing.

➡ Link up with other students who will be doing their fieldwork at the same time. Think about students from other schools or students giving up their apartments to go somewhere else.

➡ Check out local motels, youth hostels, or YMCAs/YWCAs for reasonable short-term accommodations. Often, they will give you a discount for staying consistently; or check into off-season rentals in a tourist area, such as Florida between May and November (Crist, 1996). Use your creativity and problem-solving skills to make the best situation.

I strongly recommend going away for at least one of your fieldwork experiences. It is an opportunity to explore the world, find out who you are, discover new areas in which to work and live, and learn not only how to be an OT practitioner, but also what else is out there in terms of different OT theory, state law, and practice. A student shares his experience in the following vignette:

➡ James was from a small rural town. He had never been more than 2 hours away from home. He was very anxious about going to his second site, which was located in a large metropolitan area. While there, however, he found that his values and his background helped him to relate with the patients who had come very far from home for medical treatment. He connected in a very real way and discovered that he could survive anywhere as long as he connected with people. Unless you share of yourself to help others in a meaningful way, you won't know the extent of your survival skills.

SUMMARY

Level II fieldwork is the time to develop your skills and knowledge. It is the time to extend your wings and try new things. It is the time to become the best occupational therapy practitioner that you can with the help of the mentoring process of level II fieldwork. You can always come back home, bringing new information and ideas, and work for the rest of your life. You will not find your mom or your best friend at your fieldwork site, but you will certainly find yourself. One of my favorite authors, Dr. Seuss (1990), says it best with this poem: Oh, the Places You'll Go!

"Congratulations!
Today is your day.
You're off to Great Places!
You're off and away!

You have brains in your head.
You have feet in your shoes.
You can steer yourself
any direction you choose.
You're on your own. And you know what you know.
And YOU are the guy who'll decide where to go.

...Out there things can happen and frequently do to people as brainy and footsy as you.

And when things start to happen,
Don't worry. Don't stew.
Just go right along.
You'll start happening too.

OH! THE PLACES YOU'LL GO!"

REFERENCES

Accreditation Council for Occupational Therapy Education. (1998). Standards for an accredited educational program for the occupational therapist. *Am J Occup Ther, 53, 575-582.*

American Occupational Therapy Association Conference. (2001). *Executive Director's report.* Philadelphia, PA.

Bossers, A., Cook, J., Polatajko, H., & Laine, C. (1997). Understanding the role-emerging fieldwork placement. *Can J Occup Ther, 64,* 70-81.

Commission On Education. (1999a). *Fieldwork data form.* Bethesda, MD: American Occupational Therapy Association.

Commission On Education. (1999b). *Student evaluation of fieldwork experience.* Bethesda, MD: American Occupational Therapy Association.

Crist, P. (1996). Looking for a "just right" place to live. *Advance for Occupational Therapists, 12*(32), 4.

Dunbar, S., Simhoni, O., & Anderson, L. (2001). A taxonomy of contemporary fieldwork. Education Special Interest Section Quarterly, *American Occupational Therapy Association, 11*(2), 2-4.

Herge, E., & Milbourne, S. (1999). *Self-directed learning: A model for occupational therapy fieldwork. Innovations in occupational therapy education.* Bethesda, MD: American Occupational Therapy Association.

Seuss, Dr. (1990). *Oh, the places you'll go!* New York, NY: Random House.

Chapter 7

Getting Organized

Jennifer Ruisi Cosgrove, MS, OTR

A popular home furnishings store ran an advertisement that simply says it all, "You can never be too organized." This statement is especially true for students preparing for a fieldwork experience. Occupational therapy practitioners are busier than ever. Therefore, students who get organized before a fieldwork experience begins and stay organized throughout the process will not only have a better personal experience, they will make the experience enjoyable for all involved.

By the end of this chapter, you will understand the following:

➠ The organization process for a successful fieldwork experience.

➠ The necessary supplies to have available for use during fieldwork.

➠ Various ways to maintain contact with classmates.

➠ Several of the resources available to assist with fieldwork through the American Occupational Therapy Association.

➠ The principles of time management.

➠ The steps involved with developing a personal documentation system.

What does it mean to be organized? Morgenstern (1998) suggests that organization is the process in which we create environments that encourage us to live, work, and relax. When organized, our homes, offices, and schedules allow us to be who we are and who we want to be. Developing good organizational skills is one of the key factors in functioning as a successful fieldwork student. Think back to a time when you felt unprepared for something as well as a time when you felt very prepared or pleased with your performance in something. Did organization have a role in your feelings as well as your performance in both situations? It most likely did. When we plan, prepare in advance, analyze, strategize, and attack during fieldwork placements, the experience is almost sure to be a success (Morgenstern, 1998). However, being told to get organized and wanting to get organized are two very different ways of looking at this task that awaits you.

The question you must ask yourself before beginning this process is, "Why do I want to get organized for fieldwork?" Certainly, a variety of answers may be given for this question; however, popular answers given by occupational therapy and occupational therapy assistant students may include the following:

⇒ Reduce the feeling of being overwhelmed.

⇒ Achieve more in less time.

⇒ Make better use of my talents and skills.

⇒ Increase my self-confidence.

⇒ Gain a sense of control.

⇒ Project a better image to my clients, colleagues, and fieldwork educators.

⇒ Reduce my stress, frustration, and anxiety level.

No matter what your personal reasons for getting organized may be, it is important to realize how much your professors help you with organization by providing you with a syllabus. Although the fieldwork site will provide you with objectives and an overview of expected progress during the fieldwork placement, it will not be the same level of organization that is provided to you in the academic environment. Therefore, it is necessary for everyone to do some level of fieldwork organization.

Although everyone is different in the way he or she organizes, certain strategies can and should be incorporated into a personal organization system. This chapter will give you straightforward information that you can use with little thought, including supplies to have and information to gather before starting. It will also give you information that will require reflection, including time management and personal documentation systems. Future employment positions will benefit from the development of organizational skills now. According to Kasar (2000), one of the most important professional behaviors in occupational therapy practitioners is organization. Your ability to organize will not only affect your performance as a professional, it will also affect the team you are a part of as reflected in the following statement by Kasar, "...quality and efficiency... are improved by your organizational abilities. Clients/patients and colleagues... make value assessments of the service... based on the perception of how well you are organized... how well a team performs is inherently dependent upon [its] organizational abilities..." (2000, p. 7).

It is imperative that you start getting organized now; your success as an occupational therapy practitioner depends on it.

I Just Received My Fieldwork Assignment—What Now?

The day that you have been waiting for has arrived—today, you have received your fieldwork assignment. After the initial excitement, you think, "I have plenty of time to get ready before starting." Wrong! You must begin planning right away—do not procrastinate. Planning is an important investment in fieldwork success. Planning will prepare you for the challenges that lie ahead and will ensure that you have the adequate resources. Consider practicing fieldwork organization skills during level I fieldwork.

If you fear that you are a procrastinator, you are not alone. It is estimated that 90% of college students procrastinate (Knaus, 1997). Although you may have a lot going on with your school, home, and social life, procrastinating about the fieldwork planning process will only lead to wasted time, missed opportunities, poor performance, self-depreciation, and increased stress (Keller & Heyman, 1987). Getting started in the planning process is simple. The first thing you need to do is make a phone call.

Calling the Fieldwork Site

Before you call the fieldwork site, set aside some time to think about what information is needed from the fieldwork educator at the site. Begin by viewing files kept in the fieldwork office about the site, and speak to your school's Academic Fieldwork Coordinator (AFWC) to gather as much information about the placement as you can. Inform the AFWC that you are planning to call the fieldwork site and discuss with the AFWC questions he or she recommends asking.

Although everyone will want to ask different questions and will want to know different information, it is recommended that the following information be gathered:

➠ What date would you like me to start?

➠ When can I come for an interview?

➠ What paperwork would you like to receive before I start and by what date would you like it?

➠ Will I be on a specific rotation?

➠ With what type of clients will I be involved?

➠ Who will be my direct supervisor or fieldwork educator?

➠ What are my hours?

➠ What is the dress code?

➠ What should I bring with me?

➠ Are there specific books you recommend I bring with me for reference?

➠ Can you provide me with recommended readings?

➠ Where should I park?

➠ Is it appropriate to bring or buy lunch?

➠ What advice, if any, can you give me that will help me to organize and plan for this affiliation?

➠ Should I call you again, and if so when?

Although these questions are fairly basic, they will give you foundational information to use in the planning process. Be prepared to not receive answers to all of your questions, and be aware that information provided to you may change prior to the starting date.

Designing a Plan

Take the recommendations from the fieldwork educator seriously by organizing a timeline of how you will complete the recommended readings, gather supplies, and complete the other suggestions given. Set a date to have all the necessary supplies gathered and a date to send in required paperwork. Discuss the information with family, significant others, and anyone else who will be involved with this significant change in your life. Remember that fieldwork is a completely different challenge from the typical life that you have come to know as a student in the classroom. Take the new information received to make decisions about changes that will need to take place, including moving, work responsibilities, home responsibilities, transportation, and financial issues. It may be at this time that you also talk with students or recent graduates to get their advice on how to plan for fieldwork. It is also

possible to ask your AFWC to view prior student evaluations of the fieldwork site. Finally, pat yourself on the back for taking the first few steps in getting organized for fieldwork; you have information and you have designed an initial plan. The time between finding out your placement and actually starting fieldwork is a very valuable period of time. However, as the time gets closer to your starting date, you must begin thinking about more detailed tasks that will enhance your fieldwork experience.

THE WAITING GAME

Depending upon when you receive your fieldwork assignment, you may have a significant amount of time to wait before actually beginning. However, no matter how much time you have, use it to your advantage. Continue to follow the plan you made after the initial phone call to the fieldwork educator, and begin to consider additional tasks that will make your fieldwork experience the best it can be. These tasks may include organizing a system to keep in touch with classmates by exploring and joining listservs relevant to your fieldwork site and completing your professional portfolio.

Update Initial Plan on a Regular Basis

Plan, plan, plan. Where are you with the initial plan you made after speaking with the AFWC and the fieldwork educator? Do you need to call the fieldwork educator again? Does your car need a tune-up to ensure it is in good working condition? Do you need to find housing or let a part-time job know that you will be quitting? Whatever your initial plan involved, it is important to check off accomplished tasks and continue analyzing, strategizing, and attacking on a regular basis (Morgenstern, 1998).

Analyze your initial plan, and make changes as necessary. It is critical that you get a clear picture of where you are and where you are headed. Although analyzing your organizational plan takes time to complete, it is the most important step in the organizing process. This may require completing a personal needs assessment so you have all the pertinent information available for charting a solid path to fieldwork success (Morgenstern, 1998). The needs assessment will look at what needs to be done, what has been done, what is the most important to do, and what are potential barriers to completing necessary tasks. To complete the needs assessment, record the answers to the questions in *Fieldwork Needs Assessment*.

FIELDWORK NEEDS ASSESSMENT

➡ What needs to be done to be ready for the first day of fieldwork? (Do not forget supplies, housing, transportation, finances, and studying.)

➡ What have I accomplished at this point in time?

➡ What tasks are the most important?

➡ What are potential barriers?

Next, you must strategize or create a plan of action. Assign a completion date to all of the tasks on your list, with the most important tasks having an earlier date. Pay attention to the barriers you outlined, and think about how you can keep them from interfering with your plan, thus accomplishing more in less time. Attacking your new "fieldwork to-do" list will be so much easier following the analyzing and strategizing stages. You can also feel good in knowing that your hard work ahead of time will allow you a sense of confidence and preparedness when you arrive at fieldwork on the first day.

Gather Necessary Supplies

Although gathering supplies may be a part of your new "fieldwork to-do" list, it is important and thus requires added attention. Showing up to fieldwork without the necessary supplies can cause unneeded stress. So, where are you in gathering the necessary supplies and materials the fieldwork educator outlined during your initial call? If this information was not provided, you should make your own list. This list should contain materials and supplies that you will need to bring with you on your first day of fieldwork. Here is a list of suggested supplies to have available for use during the fieldwork assignment (depending on your site, some supplies may not be applicable):

➡ This book.

➡ The fieldwork manual from your school.

➡ A nametag (include the title Occupational Therapy Student).

➡ A lab coat if appropriate.

➡ A watch with a second hand.

➡ A notebook to jot down notes.

➡ Something with which to write.

➡ Reference books.

➡ A clipboard with Handy Helper or other outlines attached (A Handy Helper is a reference sheet of useful information including manual muscle testing (MMT), range-of-motion norms, Ranchos Los Amigos Cognitive Scale, dermatomes, etc., or anything that may be of assistance to you during fieldwork).

➡ A schedule book or something to keep track of your schedule (see Time Management on p. 70).

➡ Professional portfolio.

Having these supplies prepared ahead of time shows you were reflective before the experience. This helps make the first impression a positive one.

Organize a System to Maintain Contact with Classmates

Maintaining contact with classmates while participating in fieldwork can prove to be beneficial in many ways. It is important to have a network of peers who are experiencing the same situations at the same time. Having a way to get in touch with classmates allows students to share ideas, ask for advice and support, or just have a friend at a time when one may be greatly needed. Keeping in touch may be accomplished in many ways, including developing a personal distribution list, establishing times for chat room discussions, or simply creating a classmate contact list.

One simple way to keep in touch with classmates is to create a classmate contact list. This is easily accomplished by having one person in the class circulate a form asking each person in the class to list his or her name, personal address, phone number while on fieldwork, e-mail address, and type of fieldwork. Once completed, this list should be distributed to everyone in the class. This list will allow for an instant network of friends to call on when in need of assistance or support.

Students with e-mail may choose to take the list of classmates and create a personal distribution list. A personal distribution list is a group of people to whom you can send the same e-mail to simultaneously. Creating a personal distribution list is easy and can be accomplished on most e-mail systems. If your e-mail program does not allow you to create a personal distribution list, you can still enter all the e-mail addresses of your classmates into the e-mail address book for easy reference.

Chat rooms are an excellent way to keep in touch with classmates. Before the start of a fieldwork experience, organize times and places for on-line "chats." The American Occupational Therapy Association (AOTA) has a chat room that is available 24 hours a day just for this purpose. Go to the AOTA web site at www.aota.org, and click on "chat room" under the "Highlights" area on the home page for details.

Join Listservs

While preparing for the start of a fieldwork experience, it is recommended that you begin to explore and subscribe to a listserv that is relevant to the fieldwork site. A listserv is an electronic mailing list that usually focuses on a specific topic or discipline. AOTA sponsors several listservs for occupational therapy practitioners. You must be a member of AOTA to subscribe to these listservs. As a member, you may join as many listservs as you like. Upon subscribing to a listserv, you will be able to pose questions, comments, ideas, etc., to the entire listserv as well as receive the same from other members. As a list subscriber, individuals receive copies of all e-mail sent to the listserv. Information such as this may be very beneficial to students, especially during fieldwork. When a subscriber sends an e-mail message to the listserv, a copy is e-mailed to all subscribers. For example, if you are completing a level II fieldwork in a mental health facility and you need more information for the case study on which you are working, it is possible for you to e-mail the listserv to ask the members where you may find the specific information you are looking for. AOTA has the following listservs available to its members:

➡ Administration and Management

➡ Developmental Disabilities

➡ Education

➡ Gerontology

➡ Home and Community Health

➡ Mental Health

➡ Physical Disabilities

➡ Sensory Integration

➡ School System

➡ Technology

➡ Work Programs

➡ Creativity (Discusses creative ways of problem solving and methods for increasing creativity)

➡ MDI (Multicultural Diversity and Inclusion—Discusses issues related to multicultural diversity and inclusion) (AOTA, 2001)

Listservs are a great place to share stories and ideas and to network with practitioners all over the country. For information and directions on how to subscribe to one of the many listservs offered by AOTA, consult the AOTA web site. Keep in mind that when talking with other professionals, listserv etiquette is extremely important. Use professional writing and avoid commonly held practices such as using all lower case letters, excessive smiley faces, or abbreviations.

Professional Portfolio

Finally, while waiting to begin a fieldwork placement, it is a good idea to create a professional portfolio. A professional portfolio is a compilation of various types of information about you, including personal data, academic/educational data, professional development, and fieldwork experiences. Creating a portfolio will allow you to record personal and professional growth and facilitates the self-assessment process. Some of the contents of a professional portfolio are often required during fieldwork, such as the personal data sheet, completed health forms, CPR certification, malpractice insurance policy, and health insurance certificate. Having an organized portfolio with required fieldwork data, such as the contents listed above as well as information that tells a story about you, might assist the fieldwork educator in knowing more about you. A portfolio will provide an organized way for maintaining records and documents often required during fieldwork placements. For more information on completing a professional portfolio, see Chapter 15.

FIELDWORK BEGINS

Planning, organizing, and strategizing prior to the start of fieldwork are the best ways to prepare for a successful fieldwork experience. However, staying organized while participating in fieldwork is an even greater challenge and one that will require thought and reflection. Remaining organized will involve constant examination of time management skills and the development of a personal documentation system. Reflection on your performance will also allow you to stay organized. Allowing yourself time to examine what you have or have not accomplished and how well or not so well it was accomplished usually results in thoughts about organization and changes that may be needed. Fieldwork requires you to identify your priorities and a system for accomplishing them.

Time Management

Planning, judgment, anticipation, and commitment are important components of time management (Long & McCarthy, 1997). Time management is one of the keys to success in fieldwork. It involves managing your time during and outside of the working day. Most students will find that the time management system used during the academic semester will not suffice during fieldwork. Although the time demands may seem similar, you will quickly learn that they are actually very different. The days of having hours or even weeks to study and prepare for a lab practical or class presentation are long gone. Most students will find that time in the occupational therapy practice world is much faster and at times more demanding than the academic world. As a fieldwork student, you must develop a system for living each day according to your personal priorities (Long & McCarthy, 1997).

Managing your time during fieldwork is easy to do and can assist with making the experience the best it can be. The most important way to gain control of your time is to set up a schedule. Developing a variety of schedules is important to balance your activities during the working day and after the working day and to prepare for projects requiring extensive amounts of time or activities that will, because of the time involved, take you away from your typical schedule. Successful time management comes from the creation of a master plan. During the first week of fieldwork, expectations of you and a sense of the time commitment needed should be fairly clear. At this point, it may be best to create both a monthly and weekly schedule. Following the creation of both of these, you will then be ready to create daily schedules. Creating a schedule may require purchasing a schedule book, or, if you have a computer, you may choose to use personal information management software or a spreadsheet program. Ensure that the computerized scheduling program is printable to allow for easy reference during the day or is portable, such as the popular hand-held organizers now available. Or, you may choose to make copies of the monthly, weekly, and daily schedules provided at the end of this chapter (pp. 77-79).

Effective management of your time while on fieldwork will require you to look at the 8 or 12 weeks, depending if you are an OT or OTA student, in its entirety. This can be done on a monthly block-style calendar (DiYanni, 1997). Enter the important dates you have been given by your fieldwork educator, such as in-service dates and due dates for special projects. Next, fill in activities that occur on a weekly basis that may take extra preparation time the night before, such as rounds, team meetings, and committee meetings. Finally, enter personal activities such as concert events, weddings, or any personal event that will take you away from your ability to complete fieldwork assignments. Completing a monthly calendar for the 2- or 3-month fieldwork assignment will give you a quick sense of what lies ahead of you. This long-range overview of time must be created before weekly and daily schedules can be created.

A weekly schedule requires much greater detail and thought to create. The weekly schedule must include the hours you are at fieldwork, the hours of a part-time job, home/family commitments, and time set aside for reading, studying, and working on fieldwork projects. Although it is almost always strongly recommended that students do not have a part-time job while participating in fieldwork, some students will anyway, and thus it must be included as a possible activity in your weekly schedule. The weekly schedule should also include time you need for traveling, errands, exercising, and other recreational activities. Do not forget to schedule time for fun, as recreation deserves a place in your priorities. Using the weekly schedule, it is next necessary to create a daily schedule. The daily schedule should include a very detailed listing of the hours of the day to include activities that will occur during the day at fieldwork (see *Sample Weekly Schedule* [p. 71]).

Student Activity 1

Before starting fieldwork, make a copy of the blank Weekly Schedule at the end of the chapter. Complete your schedule for the next week. At the end of the week, make note of the following:

➠ What you left out.

➠ What activities took more or less time than scheduled.

➠ The schedule's ability to keep you organized.

➠ How well you kept to the schedule.

➠ How you will use a weekly schedule to help keep you organized during fieldwork.

The daily schedule is an important tool for maintaining organization at the fieldwork site. It is a good

SAMPLE WEEKLY SCHEDULE

	Sunday	Monday	Tuesday	Wednesday	Thursday	Friday	Saturday
5:00							
6:00		Gym		Gym		Running	
7:00							
8:00		Fieldwork	Fieldwork	Fieldwork	Fieldwork	Fieldwork	
9:00							Study in library/ in-service
10:00	Part-time job						
11:00							
12:00							
1:00							
2:00							
3:00							Basketball game
4:00							
5:00		Grocery store			Dinner with Sam		
6:00	Study/set schedule						
7:00		Study/ homework	Study/ prepare for rounds	Study/work on in-service			
8:00							Movie
9:00		Watch show			Study/ homework		
10:00							
11:00							

Adapted from Long, K. F., & McCarthy, M. (1997). Time management: The foundation of academic success. In J. N. Gardner & A. J. Jewler (Eds.). *Your college experience: Strategies for success* (3rd ed., pp. 48-68). Belmont, CA: Wadsworth Publishing Company.

idea to update your daily schedule the night before, allowing for updates in treatment times, supervision times with the fieldwork educator, and planning goals for "down times." Although down times may be rare, it is important to be prepared for them if they do occur. Think about what you might like to accomplish if you suddenly had a half-hour free. Taking advantage of an unexpected half-hour may allow you to complete a literature search or gather the missing information needed for a case study project. Creating a daily schedule that is extremely detailed is imperative at the start of a fieldwork affiliation. The change from a daily student schedule to a daily fieldwork student schedule is immense. It is best to use a daily schedule that allows you to record the actual schedule kept as compared to the planned schedule. It will be difficult to keep track of the hour-to-hour and minute-to-minute requirements unless you have thought about it in advance and have planned appropriately. Once your schedule becomes a habit, the need to be so precise may decrease. Remember that it is easier to find something to do with extra time than to find extra time to do something. See *Sample Daily Schedule* (p. 73) for an example.

Student Activity 2

Before starting fieldwork, make a copy of the blank Daily Schedule form at the end of the chapter. Complete your schedule for the next day. At the end of the day, make note of the following:

➡ What you left out.

➡ What activities took more or less time than scheduled.

➡ The schedule's ability to keep you organized.

➡ How well you kept to the schedule.

➡ How you will use a daily schedule to help keep you organized during fieldwork.

Personal Documentation System

A documentation system is a system you can develop to keep track of and organize your client's progress in treatment. One of the most important functions of an occupational therapy practitioner is documentation. Because of the importance of documentation, it is imperative that it is done properly, accurately, confidentially, and in a timely fashion. Documentation will require a place or places in your daily schedule.

Documentation has many purposes including providing a profile of a client's health needs, providing the basis for a plan of care, a record of the care given and its outcome, proof of quality performance, medical research data, and protection from legal liability (Channing L. Bete Co., 2000). State, federal, and individual institutional guidelines must be taken into consideration when documenting. These guidelines, especially confidentiality, should be reviewed with you during your fieldwork orientation. However, developing your own organizational system for documentation is another way to assist you with staying organized during fieldwork. Your system for organization may include keeping a quick reference sheet about documentation on your clipboard and determining a system for remembering what was done with a client when documentation does not immediately follow intervention.

Fieldwork sites may use written or computerized charting. Whichever method, your fieldwork educator will most likely insist that he or she reviews your documentation before it is written into the chart or entered into the computerized charting system. You may be given time after each client to complete documentation, you may have a designated time during the day to complete documentation on several clients, or you may be asked to complete your documentation after you leave for the day. Because it may take you more time to complete your documentation when you first begin, your fieldwork educator may decide that it is best for you to document when you are in a quiet environment and have enough time to produce a well-written document. If your fieldwork educator asks you to do this, he or she will most likely enter his or her own documentation on the client because of the necessity to document within the time limits set by the facility. Or, your fieldwork educator may document a short note indicating that occupational therapy services were provided and that a detailed summary will be provided shortly, allowing time for you to complete the documentation on the client. In this case, it will be important for your fieldwork educator to review your notes as soon as possible—the next morning if you do your notes after the working day—so that corrections can be made and the documentation can be added to the chart as quickly as possible. Above all, it is important to remember the necessity of confidentiality when completing any documentation outside of the fieldwork site and when designing your documentation system.

Developing a Quick Reference Documentation Form

Developing a quick reference documentation form can organize the information you need for note writ-

Sample Daily Schedule

Date: Monday, June 23rd

To Do

Reschedule Mrs. Smith

Write note for Mrs. Cook

✓ Billing

✓ Speak with speech therapist re: Mr. Kelly

Call Mom

Get milk

To Look Up:

Precautions for rheumatoid arthritis

Time	Planned	Actual	Time	Planned	Actual
5:00			3:00	Mr. Kelly	Mr. Kelly
5:15			3:15		
5:30	Get up		3:30	Note	Notes
5:45		Get up	3:45	Gather info for in-service	
6:00	Gym		4:00		
6:15		Running	4:15		
6:30			4:30		
6:45			4:45		
7:00	Shower/dress	Shower/Dress	5:00	Grocery store	Store
7:15			5:15		
7:30	Travel	Travel	5:30		
7:45			5:45		
8:00	Fieldwork/organize day	Organized day	6:00	Relax	Relax
8:15			6:15		
8:30	Mrs. Smith	Observed sup.	6:30	Eat dinner	
8:45			6:45		Dinner
9:00	Mr. Jones	Mr. Jones	7:00	Study/homework	
9:15			7:15		
9:30			7:30		Study/homework
9:45	Mrs. Adams	Mrs. Adams	7:45		
10:00			8:00		
10:15			8:15		
10:30	Write notes		8:30		
10:45		Notes	8:45		
11:00	Team meeting	Team meeting	9:00	Watch TV	
11:15			9:15		TV
11:30			9:30		
11:45	Call wheelchair vendor	LM for vendor	9:45		
12:00	Lunch	Lunch	10:00	Bed	Bed
12:15			10:15		
12:30	Supervision meeting		10:30		
12:45		Sup. Meeting	10:45		
1:00	Mr. Thomas	Mr. Thomas	11:00		
1:15			11:15		
1:30	Note		11:30		
1:45	Mrs. Cook	Mrs. Cook	11:45		
2:00			12:00		
2:15			12:15		
2:30	Note	Notes	12:30		
2:45			12:45		

QUICK REFERENCE SHEET: DOCUMENTATION

RUMBA Test
Who is the audience (who will read it and who will benefit from it)?
Is it **r**elevant (does it reflect functional goals and achievement)?
Is it **u**nderstandable (is it legible, does it contain jargon)?
Is it **m**easurable (do goals and statements include frequency and duration)?
Is it **b**ehavioral (document behaviors not descriptors of attitude)?
Is it **a**chievable (is the goal realistic)?

SOAP Notes:
Subjective (S)—the client's perception of the intervention being received, progress, limitations, needs, and problems.
Objective (O)—your observations of the intervention being provided as well as the observable and measurable data.
Assessment (A)—your interpretation of the information reported in the objective section. Also include functional limitations and your expectations for the client to benefit from intervention.
Plan (P)—what you plan to have the patient do next in order to work toward the goals set.

Adapted from Perinchief, J. M. (1998). Management of occupational therapy services. In M. E. Neistadt & E. B. Crepeau (Eds.), *Willard & Spackman's occupational therapy* (pp. 783-787). Philadelphia, PA: Lippincott-Raven Publishers and Borcherding, S. (2000). *Documentation manual for writing SOAP notes in occupational therapy.* Thorofare, NJ: SLACK Incorporated.

---

ing. For example, you may want a list of questions to ask yourself during and after writing. You may also want to list reminders about the documentation that is required by the facility, such as a guide for writing SOAP (standing for Subjective, Objective, Assessment, and Plan) notes. Whatever you determine as important for keeping you organized while documenting is important to list on your quick reference sheet (see *Quick Reference Sheet: Documentation*).

According to Perinchief (1998), the following questions may assist in organizing the thought process in approaching documentation:

⟹ Who is the audience (who will read it and who will benefit from it)?

⟹ Is it **r**elevant (does the documentation reflect functional goals and achievement)?

⟹ Is it **u**nderstandable (is it legible, does it contain jargon)?

⟹ Is it **m**easurable (do goals and statements include frequency and duration)?

⟹ Is it **b**ehavioral (document behaviors not descriptors of attitude)?

⟹ Is it **a**chievable (is the goal realistic)?

Hopefully, you noticed the acronym RUMBA from the above questions. The RUMBA test can be used to assess documentation. Adding the RUMBA test to a documentation quick reference sheet may assist you as you complete documentation at the fieldwork site.

A popular patient-centered approach to documentation is the SOAP note. The SOAP format is an alternative to narrative notes, which tend to be disorganized and subjective (Borcherding, 2000). Even though you have practiced writing SOAP notes in various classes, prior learning is often difficult to recall when in new and possibly stressful situations like a fieldwork site. It is recommended that you add the components of a SOAP note to your quick reference sheet for times when you need a gentle reminder. The following description of the components of a SOAP note is adapted from Borcherding (2000):

⟹ Subjective (S)—the client's perception of the intervention being received, progress, limitations, needs, and problems.

⟹ Objective (O)—your observations of the intervention being provided as well as the observable and measurable data.

⟹ Assessment (A)—your interpretation of the information reported in the objective section. Also include functional limitations and your expectations for the client to benefit from intervention.

⟹ Plan (P)—what you plan to have the patient do next in order to work toward the goals set.

Recording Personal Notes

As was previously stated, you may not have the option to complete documentation immediately following a session with a client. Because of the importance of accurate documentation, students participating in fieldwork should develop a system to briefly record personal notes about a session for later reference. Keeping these notes organized and confidential is most important. Therefore, use the initials of the client in your documentation; never record the full name of a client. You may choose to keep your notes in a small notebook or on your personal clipboard. However, mobile computing technology, such as the Palm Pilot, is also an acceptable way to document information for later reference. Mobile computing technology has the advantage of assisting with maintaining confidentiality but the downside of requiring more time to record, especially for users new to the technology. Include the following information in your personal documentation:

➠ Time session started and ended.

➠ What was done during the session.

➠ Client's performance/reactions.

➠ Other pertinent information you may later forget.

Taking just a minute or two to jot down a few notes will assist with completing a well-written and accurate note later in the day.

Client Log

At the completion of your fieldwork experience, you will be asked to complete the Student Evaluation of Fieldwork Experience form from the AOTA (2000). The purpose of this evaluation is to provide feedback about your fieldwork experience to your faculty and other students in your occupational therapy program as well as to your fieldwork educator and the fieldwork facility. This form will require you to comment on the types of assignments required, clients on your caseload, and types of interventions you performed during your fieldwork experience. It is recommended that you keep an organized running log of this information during the fieldwork experience. This will assist with completing the form at the end and will also allow you to reflect back on the many different experiences that your fieldwork placement allowed you (see *Fieldwork Data Log* on p 76).

Reflection on Your Performance

One final suggestion for maintaining organization during your fieldwork experience is to allow time for reflection on your performance. Although you have probably had experience in keeping a journal to reflect on your clinical reasoning and observational skills in school, it is a good idea to reflect on your organizational skills as well. Every time we go through a major change like starting fieldwork, we experience a breakdown in our organizational systems. This breakdown is inevitable because you are dealing with a new set of realities and it takes time to process the information and see clearly what and how to keep organized (Morgenstern, 1998). Being reflective about your performance as well as your ability to remain organized is easily accomplished by completing a journal in the form of a weekly progress report. This self-evaluative report can also be shared with your fieldwork educator during weekly supervision meetings. The weekly progress report will be extremely helpful in keeping you organized with developing weekly plans and goals (see *Weekly Progress Report* on p. 77).

CONCLUSION

This chapter has attempted to assist occupational therapy students with organizational skills necessary for a successful fieldwork experience. Getting organized before and staying organized during a fieldwork experience is essential. Taking the time to design various organizational plans and reflecting on those plans will lead to a feeling of internal organization that is seen externally as a meritorious quality by fieldwork educators and other members of the team.

REFERENCES

American Occupational Therapy Association. (2001). AOTA listservs. Retrieved March 25, 2002, from http://www.aota.org.

American Occupational Therapy Association, Commission on Education, Fieldwork Issues Committee. (2000). *Student evaluation of fieldwork experience.* Bethesda, MD: Author.

Borcherding, S. (2000). *Documentation manual for writing SOAP notes in occupational therapy.* Thorofare, NJ: SLACK Incorporated.

Channing L. Bete Co., Inc. (2000). *Documenting patient care to meet JCAHO standards* [Brochure]. South Deerfield, MA: Author.

DiYanni, R. (1997). *How to succeed in college.* Needham Heights, MA: Allyn and Bacon.

Kasar, J. (2000). The meaning of professionalism. In J. Kasar & E. N. Clark (Eds.), *Developing professional behaviors.* Thorofare, NJ: SLACK Incorporated.

FIELDWORK DATA LOG

Keep track of the number of times you perform the following activities. It may be best to update the list weekly to ensure accuracy.
- ⟹ Client/Patient Screening:
- ⟹ Client/Patient Evaluations (include specific names of evaluations):
- ⟹ Written Treatment/Care Plans:
- ⟹ Discharge Summary:
- ⟹ Team Meeting Presentations:
- ⟹ In-service Presentations (include titles):
- ⟹ Case Study (include title):
- ⟹ Quality/Outcome/Efficacy Study:
- ⟹ Activity Analysis:
- ⟹ Supervision of Aides, OTAs, Level I Students, and Volunteers:
- ⟹ Other:

Caseload Description: (attach additional sheets as needed)

Client Initials	Age	Condition/ Problem	Major Therapeutic Interventions Used

Adapted from American Occupational Therapy Association. Commission on Education, Fieldwork Issues Committee. (2000). *Student evaluation of fieldwork experience*. Bethesda, MD: Author.

Keller, P. A., & Heyman, S. R. (1987). *Innovations in clinical practice: A source book* (Vol. 6). Sarasota, FL: Professional Resource Exchange, Inc.

Knaus, W. J. (1997). *Do it now: Break the procrastination habit.* New York, NY: John Wiley and Sons.

Long, K. F., & McCarthy, M. (1997). Time management: The foundation of academic success. In J. N. Gardner & A. J. Jewler (Eds.), *Your college experience: Strategies for success* (3rd ed.). Belmont, CA: Wadsworth Publishing Company.

Morgenstern, J. (1998). *Organizing from the inside out.* New York, NY: Henry Holt and Company, LLC.

Perinchief, J. M. (1998). Management of occupational therapy services. In M. E. Neistadt & E. B. Crepeau (Eds.), *Willard & Spackman's occupational therapy.* Philadelphia, PA: Lippincott-Raven Publishers.

WEEKLY PROGRESS REPORT: A PERSONAL REFLECTION

Date: _____   Week #: _____

The past week was _____

Strengths and difficulties with screening and evaluation:

Strengths and difficulties with intervention:

Strengths and difficulties with discharge and transition planning:

Strengths and difficulties with documentation and communication:

Strengths and difficulties with organizational skills:

Personal goals for the next week:

Month: _____

Sunday	Monday	Tuesday	Wednesday	Thursday	Friday	Saturday

Monthly schedule form.

	Sunday	Monday	Tuesday	Wednesday	Thursday	Friday	Saturday
5:00							
6:00							
7:00							
8:00							
9:00							
10:00							
11:00							
12:00							
1:00							
2:00							
3:00							
4:00							
5:00							
6:00							
7:00							
8:00							
9:00							
10:00							
11:00							

Weekly schedule form.

Date: _____

	Planned	Actual		Planned	Actual	To Do
5:00			3:00			
5:15			3:15			
5:30			3:30			
5:45			3:45			
6:00			4:00			
6:15			4:15			
6:30			4:30			
6:45			4:45			
7:00			5:00			
7:15			5:15			
7:30			5:30			
7:45			5:45			
8:00			6:00			
8:15			6:15			
8:30			6:30			To Look Up:
8:45			6:45			
9:00			7:00			
9:15			7:15			
9:30			7:30			
9:45			7:45			
10:00			8:00			
10:15			8:15			
10:30			8:30			
10:45			8:45			
11:00			9:00			
11:15			9:15			
11:30			9:30			
11:45			9:45			
12:00			10:00			
12:15			10:15			
12:30			10:30			
12:45			10:45			
1:00			11:00			
1:15			11:15			
1:30			11:30			
1:45			11:45			
2:00			12:00			
2:15			12:15			
2:30			12:30			
2:45			12:45			

Daily schedule form.

Chapter 8

WORK ALL DAY, HOMEWORK ALL EVENING

Brenda Smaga, MS, OTR, FAOTA

Fieldwork has unique stages that educators often informally call the *honeymoon*, the *copycat*, the *know-it-all*, and the *juggler stages*. In this chapter, learning opportunities are explored for these unique stages of fieldwork. By understanding what happens at each stage, you will be able to understand their role in mastering learning expectation, including how to do the following:

➡ Use the fieldwork stages to your benefit.

➡ Master those projects.

➡ Think creatively.

➡ Develop client relationships.

➡ Feel comfortable and improve confidence.

➡ Avoid communication mishaps.

➡ Master using resources appropriately.

➡ Cotreat effectively.

➡ Apply academic knowledge to clinical settings.

STAGE I—HONEYMOON

Fieldwork has a natural flow to it, and at every turning point, there are new opportunities for molding yourself into the practitioner you want to become. You may look forward with anticipation and excitement mixed with some fear and anxiety before you begin, but the first several weeks are definitely the most exhilarating. It starts with the "honeymoon" stage, a time when you see new procedures and confirmation of those you learned in your classes. You will say to yourself, "I learned that," "I can do that." Most of your learning at this stage is through observation, as your fieldwork educator evaluates and treats clients, some of whom will eventually be yours to treat.

This is a time to regroup and review academic work that is directly related to what you are observing, such as terminology used on the evaluations or the precautions needed when doing specific treatments. If there is an evaluation that you have never seen before, this is the time to study the manual and endeavor to learn the basics of the protocol. When you observe the therapist doing it again, you will feel more able to do it yourself later.

Another opportunity that you will have at this stage, but not a chance to do later, is to know your clients informally. Developing a relationship will help you feel more comfortable with your role as the student, given that most clients love to share and teach students themselves. Your clients can educate you in all manners of things, such as what the individual therapies are doing for them, how they feel about their stage in life, and what their normal occupations are. Using the suggestions in *Know Those Therapies!* (p. 83), develop a survey to understand client perspective.

Many students wonder about asking questions and to whom. Most will gravitate toward the person they see as most willing and encouraging. This may not always be your clinical supervisor. Focus on developing a balance, as staff relationships are usually well formed before you have arrived on the scene, and your goal is to fit in, not alienate. If you feel you are asking too many questions, you may be accurate. This should be a clue that you need lots more information on this topic, rather than clarifying a few points. Another way to get needed information is to write these questions in your journal and look for resources in the clinic or in your textbooks that might answer them just as well.

At the end of this stage, feelings of anxiousness may arise, knowing that the "observation" period is over and you are expected to perform the tasks you have been observing. How best to avoid panic at this time is to be sure from the very first day that you have been interacting with your clients and doing small parts of the procedures, giving you hands-on experiences. If you find yourself standing back, not interacting, not asking to assist, not touching the client, you may be headed for a panic attack on the day the therapist asks you to do it yourself (Hall, 2001).

In summary, what have you learned in the "honeymoon" stage? You should now have perfected your observation skills, have explored where the learning resources are in this facility, have formed relationships with clients, and feel confident you know the learning expectations for the evaluation, treatment, and documentation procedures in this facility. Review the reflective questions in *How Do I Get My Questions Answered?* (p. 83), *Could This Happen To You—Friendly or Frozen?* (p. 83), and *Which Is Your Style—Germane or Irrelevant?* (p. 84) to see how others addressed honeymoon issues.

STAGE II—COPYCAT

The next stage of fieldwork is the "copycat" stage. This is the stage that will teach you to do the essential job functions of the OT or OTA. You now want to learn the fundamentals of what your therapist does every day. How do you accomplish this? In this stage, your supervisor will assign clients that are the most typical in the caseload and probably need evaluations and treatment that are most commonly done at this facility. In the therapist's mind, they will also be the easiest to treat, to transfer, and with whom to communicate. You will still be observing your supervisor treat so that you can initially use procedures that he or she uses to treat your client. Learning at this stage is accomplished by doing, doing, doing. Performance skills are the major learning method. Repetition is key. How many stand pivot transfers you do will translate into competence. You need all the practice you can get. Using student colleagues and family members becomes indispensable.

After your supervisor observes you doing a procedure, the feedback you are seeking is, "Am I doing this correctly?" Each time you do the procedure, it should feel more routine and more comfortable. It is normal to initially feel self-conscious and anxious when the therapist is observing you, rather than the other way around. You may find it helpful to talk your way through each task you are performing. This will help your client know exactly what you want done and will also let your supervisor know when you need help. In this stage, informational questions should be saved for your weekly supervision session or after the treatment session. During treatment, your interactions

KNOW THOSE THERAPIES!

The honeymoon stage is the time to explore what other therapies do. Later, when you cotreat, you will be happy to have had at least one observation of your client being treated by another therapy. Interdisciplinary roles and responsibilities vary in each facility. Is it only the speech therapist who performs oral-motor stimulation? Does the PT or OT measure and order the wheelchair? To understand who performs what in your facility, develop interview questions that you can use when meeting the therapists. Then, develop a set of questions for your client that will aid you in understanding his or her perspective, and interview him or her, too. This is one arena that may cause students concern as they ponder why some clients get therapies and others do not. So, have your questions ready, and do not forget to add your own reflections in your fieldwork journal during fieldwork.

HOW DO I GET MY QUESTIONS ANSWERED?

Sometimes, students get stuck and take the easy way out by always asking someone for the information they want whether it is the definition of a simple term or the more complicated procedures. Most supervisors are looking for their students to take initiative and search for information from various sources, not just from textbooks. Brainstorm on all the sources you may have available to you during fieldwork. Do not forget to include on your list other students on fieldwork from other schools or your clients.

COULD THIS HAPPEN TO YOU—FRIENDLY OR FROZEN?

Marie was a quiet and shy person. She was very studious and did well in her classes but did not like to be called on in class. Her first fieldwork with children was a dream. She loved it. The second one scared her to death. She was always afraid she would do something wrong, so during client treatment she constantly asked her fieldwork educator questions or for help. Soon, her clients lost confidence in her ability to treat them and refused to have her. She was well into her fourth week when she ended the fieldwork in tears. When asked to relate the strategies she used for dealing with her increasing anxiety, she vacillated back and forth between two dead-end strategies. First, she blamed the supervisor, even though she said she was a good supervisor. Her second strategy was to keep plugging away, hoping it would get better. This reminds one of Hem and Haw who arrived at Cheese Station C expecting to find their cheese even though it was gone the day before. They, too, complained that this should not happen to them and they were "entitled" to their cheese. So, every day, Hem and Haw went to the cheese station, found no cheese, then returned home carrying their worries and frustrations with them (Johnson, 1998). Dealing with anxiety in the honeymoon stage is crucial. Left unattended, it will grow and immobilize as more responsibilities are added. Some anxiety is normal and even spurs on someone to try something new. Students should be able to recognize their beginning achievements and gain confidence in this first stage. If not, they will stay "frozen," still looking for their "cheese" that has long since moved.

with the supervisor should be "how" questions such as, how much, how often, or how firm to touch.

In the copycat stage, the therapist's primary concern is how safe you are with clients. If you are not being given the privilege to treat independently during this stage, it is probably due to his or her unease about your attention to safety. This is the stage in which it is a necessity to review safety procedures at home and ask yourself, "Am I doing this in a safe manner?" every time you do something with a client.

Just one unsafe move, and you will find yourself under the microscope for the rest of your fieldwork.

At this stage of learning, you will not only learn the tasks, but it is essential to learn how to grade an activity and when to change a treatment activity to another one. This can be a pitfall for some students who are so anxious to do it the "correct" way that they forget that each person needs a somewhat different approach from the last client. Each time you see a client, there will be changes from the time before.

WHICH IS YOUR STYLE—GERMANE OR IRRELEVANT?

Do you want to know how to drive your fieldwork educator crazy? Connie had it perfected, but she did not even realize the effect she was having. Connie asked a million questions of her supervisor, and many of them were irrelevant to what they were doing. In fact, she asked seemingly random questions such as, "Why is that toy car in this room?" In class, she interrupted others and was the first one to raise her hand. Her peers got tired of her "know-it-all" attitude. Her clinical supervisor reported to the academic fieldwork coordinator (AFWC) that she was exhausted answering these questions. Another student had a similar affect. Judith talked incessantly, and much of it was irrelevant. For her, it was just a nervous habit, and because fieldwork initially made her nervous, she talked and talked and talked. The clients loved it, but the supervisor and other staff quickly tired of it. Judith's supervisor had the perfect solution. She just did not answer her, not even a word. So if you are getting the silent treatment, maybe it is time to look at the effect you are having on others and begin to use alternative strategies to deal with those frazzled nerves.

They might not feel well or be weaker, stronger, less interested, agitated, or even angry. Being flexible and prepared to grade the activity on the spot to meet your client's current needs is another skill to learn at this stage. For students treating young clients, I often hear about the hours of preparation for the five or six different activities they will do in the half-hour of treatment. This intense planning and preparation is a large part of the "evening's homework." At this stage, another part of evening preparation will be several projects or case studies due at the end of fieldwork. This is a good time to choose from the suggested projects in *Not More Homework!* (p. 85) and begin outlining what you want to do. Look at *Risks of Working an Outside Job or Taking a Course During Fieldwork* (p. 85) for other good reasons for not working or taking extra courses during fieldwork.

When you are trying so hard to learn to do the procedures, you may feel frustrated when you learn that your supervisor wants you to do them differently than you were taught at school. Now you ask yourself, "What is the correct way to do this?" and "Who is right—the therapist or the professor?" There are varieties of ways to do most of the treatment procedures in occupational therapy, and all may be viable. So, do not look to blame the supervisor or the professor for pulling the rug out from under you. Just learn the new procedure and be happy you are exposed to diverse ways. It will help you develop your skills of clinical reasoning by acknowledging the many theories that you can call upon to decide what to do with a client.

At the end of this stage, the midterm of your fieldwork experience, you should be able to write a list of treatment, evaluation, and documentation procedures that you feel comfortable and competent to do. This list should include such things as particular evaluations,

standard transfer techniques, progress notes, team meetings, and client and staff interactions. From this list, you will be able to set learning goals for the next stage of fieldwork that will focus on more difficult procedures and include experiences in which you are especially interested. *Would You Do This—Work or Entertain?* (p. 86) demonstrates the need to develop learning goals.

STAGE III—KNOW-IT-ALL

The next stage of fieldwork is daunting. Just when you think you should be seeing the light at the end of the tunnel, it dawns upon you that there is so much to learn and so little time in which to do it. You ask yourself, "How will I ever be able to know all that my supervisor knows?" This is a scary feeling, and you will not be able to know all that he or she knows. Forget that idea. There are more important things to focus on in this "know-it-all " stage.

Now that you feel comfortable with most of the hands-on experiences, it will be easier to expand your learning repertoire to include those more difficult procedures and evaluations. Your supervisor will add cases in which there are more difficult transfers, more complicated safety issues, clients with multiple serious illnesses, and those with whom communication may be limited. You will probably find yourself again seeking out resources, but this time you will look in different places than just your textbooks. This may require a search for a specialized text or an article on current research in the field. It is also a good time to seek out your colleagues from school, both professors and your classmates who might have treated clients with these problems. Listserv resources (see *Listserv for Communication and Collaboration* on p. 86) might be helpful.

Not More Homework!

Each of your fieldwork sites will likely schedule you to do at least two projects or presentations. This is when you know you do not want to have an outside job during fieldwork. Your success is dependent on how relevant you make them to your own personal growth and in meeting the needs of the facility. The most typical assignments are a case study and an activity analysis. However, there are lots more that you can suggest, too.

Does this facility have a student manual? You would be the best person to develop a pleasing-to-the-eye student manual that would have everything a student needs to know about this facility.

Does the nursing staff need an in-service on wheelchair safety for the clients in the geri-psych unit? This gives you a chance to use previously learned information with the focus on presentation and teaching to another discipline. Perhaps you would prefer to perform an evidence-based practice review on a rehab-related topic that you recently observed and present it to the rehabilitation department during their regular in-service. In-service presentations should use an interactive approach, include opportunity for questions and comments, and include presentation aids when possible.

Community site visits give you the opportunity to explore other areas of clinical practice as well as community resources. Would you like to see what the competition is doing? How about personally knowing where your clients are discharged? Networking for a future job may be your motivation for exploring a new place. When presenting or writing about your visit, include the relevant background information, as well as such program information as philosophy, services offered, physical facilities, disciplines and roles of staff, and population served. Do not forget to include your impressions.

If you are creative, there are lots of projects you can make and give to the facility for use with future clients. Now is the time to look at all those resource manuals you assembled for class and all those projects you labored over and see if your facility could use any. These may include a fun sensory stimulation bag of tricks for children or a game to create opportunities for practicing better judgment using stimulating questions on a deck of cards and a child's game board such as Chutes and Ladders. Would you like to construct a wooden body puzzle for body scheme or a maze that accommodates a light ping-pong ball that can be used to increase finger extension? The sky is the limit in this area. Relevancy, though, is the key.

If you have constructed an assistive technology device or a special splint for a client, think about making this your project. In this case, the relevancy is to the immediate client, but you can expand it into an educational presentation for others. Showing the steps in construction, research about the materials, their safety, and similar products makes this interesting for staff who want to explore using new materials. Cover all bases in your presentation by using the Human Activity Assistive Technology model as a guide (Cook & Hussey, 1995).

Developing a brochure or booklet for client education is a superb and relevant project. Include photos or drawings to illustrate a concept or the correct procedure. You can try your prototype with your client and then perfect it for others to use with their clients.

Whatever you decide to do, remember the key is relevancy coupled with your special interest.

Risks of Working an Outside Job or Taking a Course During Fieldwork

Most AFWCs will tell you to never work or take a course during fieldwork. This is excellent advice but might not be possible for every student. However, if you are one of the few who must work or take a course, be aware of the consequences so you can adjust your work or study schedule if needed.

Fieldwork educators of working students complain that students come to fieldwork tired, inattentive, slow moving, unenthusiastic, and unable to learn without repeated directions. They say such students are late with assignments and have an increased number of absences. If the student cannot make adjustments and improve in these areas, he or she is usually asked to leave.

Usually, students taking a course are doing so to finish graduation requirements. This is easy to prevent by taking the time needed to meet with your advisor and review your program requirements each semester. Some students who transfer credit wait until the last minute and may get a surprise notice that they need another course to complete a requirement. The conflict with fieldwork will come in juggling nightly fieldwork assignments with course assignments, causing late nights.

RISKS OF WORKING AN OUTSIDE JOB OR TAKING A COURSE DURING FIELDWORK (CONTINUED)

If you must work, it should be restricted to weekends and never more than 12 hours of work per week. Keeping 1 day a week free for relaxation and family time is beneficial. It is extremely tiring to work 7 days a week for 8 to 12 weeks. Working during the week usually causes the most problems. The type of work will affect the outcome, too, so be aware of work that is physically tiring.

In all cases, once you have been confronted with fieldwork concerns about your behavior, making rapid adjustments to decrease your work or study schedule is essential.

WOULD YOU DO THIS—WORK OR ENTERTAIN?

After lunch, the supervisor told Ken that they will be treating a patient with a work-related injury and will be using the work simulator with that client. Because this equipment is computer based and has many attachments for simulating job tasks, the supervisor informed the student that he should spend the afternoon experimenting with it and then they could plan the client's treatment when they met at 3:30 pm for supervision. The fieldwork educator was scheduled to treat outpatients in the clinic upstairs. Ken asked if he could observe her treating outpatients for a while. That seemed fine with the supervisor. However, the student stayed until 3:00 pm and, on the way back, announced to the supervisor that he wanted to stop and see the unit that was just newly renovated. Ken met his supervisor at 3:30 pm and was excited about what he observed, but was unprepared to plan tomorrow's treatment. Sometimes there are so many exciting learning opportunities, students forget the purpose of fieldwork. Becoming entry-level competent in a particular area of practice takes concentrated effort, repetitive experiences, and a focused learning plan. As a fieldwork student, you are there to learn, not to be entertained by fun and unique experiences.

LISTSERV FOR COMMUNICATION AND COLLABORATION

Computers and the web now offer more avenues for communications. One of these is to develop a listserv that is for you and your classmates to discuss your concerns and share information while you are in the fieldwork semester. There are several ways that you can do this. Your professor might be using a "classroom" program such as WebCT, Blackboard.com, or Manhattan Project that allows chatrooms and discussion bulletin boards for student groups.

If this is not available, there are several free commercial sites that allow you to create a listserv that incorporates the ability to post e-mails to the group, have a chat discussion, and attach files in your "resource" room. http://groups.yahoo.com is one such place. This requires that one person in your group be the "manager" and add or delete e-mail addresses as people change theirs. Your group is given an e-mail address, such as fieldwork@groups.yahoo.com. Then every member of the group can e-mail the whole group using this address unique to your group.

The most basic method is to create an e-mail "group" using your e-mail program, such as Outlook Express. In this case, you put everyone's e-mail address in a group list and then you e-mail the list itself to each member so they can create their own group list in their e-mail programs. Give your group list a name, such as Fieldwork. Then, when anyone sends an e-mail to this group list, the whole group gets it. However, if someone changes his or her e-mail address, everyone has to make sure that he or she changes the group list or some people will not get future messages. This is where everyone has to act as the "manager."

Lots of students like to use the reply button to send their new message, but be aware that the discussion thread may get confusing. Some student e-mail addresses will not give you much of a clue of who they are, so unless you want to memorize everyone's address, it is best to add your signature to your e-mail. Be forewarned that this is not a good method for sending personal information, as everyone receives the e-mail and all the replies. As a group, establish a list of listserv etiquette. Develop and practice professional skills on your listserv.

Treating complicated cases puts you in a great learning situation. Many facilities encourage co-treatment and collaboration. This approach requires a major switch in your thinking. In the classroom, borrowing ideas from each other at times would have been called *cheating*. In the clinic, it is considered a necessity, and if you do not do it, your supervisor will think you are not open to learning new things. Collaboration is the means of learning in this "know-it-all" stage. This is no time to be shy. Now everyone treating the client is asking questions and throwing out possible ideas. All the team members are searching for answers by exploring their collective experiences with past cases and looking at current research. Your active participation will help you feel more of an equal member of the team and will prepare you for the next stage of fieldwork.

In addition to the more challenging cases, learning will focus on analysis, synthesis, and decision making. All those clinical reasoning processes that you learned in class will help you make decisions about what to evaluate, how to treat, and when to discharge. For example, you may now feel very comfortable administrating the Kohlman Evaluation of Living Skills (KELS) and scoring it. But can you interpret what it means for your client? How will the results influence your decision about what treatment to use with your client? Your supervisor is making these decisions every day, many times a day, and when you get to this fieldwork stage, you will begin to notice the importance of this skill. A common student concern is how to see the forest for the trees. In the copycat stage, you were intently looking at the trees, and rightfully so. Now, you need to learn to let the performance skills routinely flow, so you can focus your energy on developing your decision-making skills. This is the stage to review the course material on clinical reasoning outlined in Chapter 13. Take each part of your client's problems, and examine them by writing your thoughts as you would a diagnostic decision tree. With the limited time to treat, remember to prioritize and keep it simple in the beginning. You will now be competent to write treatment goals and objectives.

You cannot approach fieldwork acting "empty headed," as though you have learned nothing at school (Crist, 1997). The fund of knowledge you bring with you from your college courses will aid you at this stage. If you do not have that knowledge base, you will be guessing all over the place. Your confidence will take a nosedive, and you will blame all your professors for not teaching you what you need to know or the supervisor for not telling you the answer. This is

when it really dawns on you that you are the only person responsible for your learning. Unless you are extremely charming and good at bluffing, this could be a major pitfall. How to avoid this? Study, study, study. *Would You Really Say This—Diplomatic or Foolhardy?* (p. 88) gives examples of statements students have made to their supervisors that may preclude success. Explore these and some of the suggested scenarios in *Group Discussion Activity: Is This Really Happening?* (p. 88) using a group format to discover various options.

Another measurement of a successful student is his or her ability to think creatively. What does this mean? In the copycat stage, you used many of the same treatment procedures and activities that your supervisor did, but with grading and modifications. In this stage, you will be responsible for designing your own activities. It is important to recognize that there is no "cookbook" to tell you what activity to do with what patient. Even so, students will spend an inordinate amount of time looking for one instead of relying on their own excellent ideas. You may ask yourself, "How am I supposed to dream up these activities?" Reviewing the treatment goals and objectives should be your starting place. Next, look at the successful occupations that your client has enjoyed in the past or those that he or she will need to do in the future. If your client actually performs this former or needed occupation, will your client meet some of the treatment objectives? What can you add or do to make this activity more stimulating, fun, interactive, successful, and unique? Does it have enough repetition to give the practice the client needs to master the objective? Can you grade its complexity as your client changes his or her ability to do it? As with all "designing," revisit what you have fashioned several times to refine it and to be sure the activity as you plan to present it will meet your client's needs.

At the "know-it-all" stage, you are learning new treatment procedures that are more detailed and complex, and the same will be true of the documentation. You will find that your writing has picked up speed and you are now putting your notes directly in the client's record. During this stage, it is a good time to schedule and complete fieldwork visits to other sites, work on special projects, and attend in-services offered at your facility.

In summary, at this stage, you do "know it all"—well, at least as much as you will need to be a beginning therapist. You have mastered the evaluation, treatment, and documentation procedures as well as having experienced many more complex issues.

WOULD YOU REALLY SAY THIS—DIPLOMATIC OR FOOLHARDY?

When Jen was having problems, the AFWC was called and asked to meet with the student and the fieldwork educator. The fieldwork educator had asked Jen, an OTA student, to do a functional muscle test on a client. Jen said she never learned this in class. The AFWC reminded her of the class and how this was taught. "Oh, yeah, I remember that now," Jen said. That fieldwork setting never accepted another student from this school.

Ashley told her fieldwork educator on the first day of fieldwork that she was going back to school and never intended to practice as an OTA. Ashley could not understand why the fieldwork educator looked at her with annoyance some of the time.

Kathy complained to her classmates that her fieldwork educator was working her to death. She told her fieldwork educator that she was exhausted and not used to this type of schedule. Her fieldwork educator related how she worked full-time when she went to college full-time.

Julie told her OTA fieldwork educator that she really wanted to be an OT and asked if she could spend more time with the OT and not as much with her. After the fieldwork educator discussed this with the OT fieldwork educator, they both agreed to limit the student's contact with the OT.

Marty thought his fieldwork educator was a dummy and complained to the rehab supervisor that he was not learning anything and wanted to change fieldwork educators. His request was denied, and his workload was increased.

Tia was the first to enter the room for a team meeting and later told her fieldwork educator, "You were late." The fieldwork educator seemed to find fault with her every action after that time.

Carolyn wanted to do a project, not a case study. She argued with her fieldwork educator who told her to do the case study. Carolyn stated that both were choices given in the student handbook for the facility. The fieldwork educator replied, "I wrote the handbook and you will do the case study."

In the classroom setting, students might say something that annoys the professor, too, such as "Should I study this? Will it be on the test? I enjoyed the demo but will a real therapist do it that way, too?" However, the consequences for the student are far different in the clinical setting. In this one-on-one relationship, the fieldwork educator and student spend 40 hours a week together. First impressions are formed by these types of comments and often get things off to a poor start, some never to fully recover.

GROUP DISCUSSION ACTIVITY: IS THIS REALLY HAPPENING?

There are small incidents that happen in fieldwork that students feel are only happening to them. These issues actually come to light rather often, and you are not alone. Explore them before beginning fieldwork by asking your AFWC to put some on cards. Sitting in a circle in class, each group member picks one and takes a guess as to how he or she would handle the situation. Then, ask the other group members to contribute their own ideas. Some of these could be: "My supervisor asked me to treat Theresa, and I never met her before." "My supervisor has a habit of asking me to stay late without much warning, and I have to pick my children up from day care." "The OT student thinks that because I am an OTA student, I should do all the cleanup." "I never eat lunch with the other OT staff." "The other student I do a group with on Wednesdays wants me to plan it each time." "A client tried to grab my arm and kiss it." "My client told me, 'I do not want to be treated today. Go away.'"

STAGE IV—JUGGLER

The "juggler" stage is the last, but shortest, stage of fieldwork. During these last few weeks of fieldwork, you are carrying a full case load and zooming around trying to complete the finishing touches on your project or presentation due any day. At this time, your major learning experience is having at least 80% to 100% of your supervisor's cases to evaluate and treat with indirect supervision. This is a real test of your ability to juggle different responsibilities, knowing that

How Should You Respond—Building or Burning Your Bridges?

Bernadette was frustrated with her fieldwork educator. Her fieldwork educator was not motivated or interested in her job and let Bernadette treat all her cases from week 3. Sometimes, she just did not show up for work and left instructions for what Bernadette should do.

Sarah's fieldwork educator and two other rehab staff members quit their jobs on the unit she was assigned to about 2 weeks after she arrived. She and another student on the same unit teamed up and tried to lead the groups and community outings in this mental health facility. The OT program supervisor would meet with them every morning to provide as much supervision as she could, but could not attend nor observe their groups because of her other responsibilities.

Jean came to her facility one day in her seventh week to find her fieldwork educator gone. She was not sure why, but could tell her leaving was not on good terms. Although others pitched in, she was left a lot on her own.

Dave was trying as hard as he could to pass his clinical. Dave was asked to stay another 2 weeks because he just could not seem to put it all together. The facility seemed to bend over backwards to make sure he succeeded. At the end, his fieldwork educator gave him passing, but low, scores in most areas. Dave was devastated and angry. He wanted to write a letter saying how mean his fieldwork educator was and that she should not have students.

All these students shared a common concern. They were worried about their education. Would they learn all that they needed to pass the certification exam and be able work independently? They were angry, too. They felt cheated and wanted to use the evaluation form that students complete to give feedback to the facility to vent their anger. Venting your anger to your closest friend, your family, or your pet dog will help put things in perspective. There are lots of strategies to use to make these placements successful, but complaining, blaming, and writing negative letters will only make things worse.

First, assess your situation and make a mental note of the people within the facility whom you could possibly have as mentors. Next, remember that, in fieldwork, your clients and your own participation provide you with most of your learning experiences. Evaluate in what activities you can participate that will give you good learning experience. Maybe attending the multiple sclerosis (MS) clinic once a week will add to your knowledge even if this was not in the original plan. Then, call your AFWC, discuss your ideas, and refine your strategies together. At your next meeting with the program supervisor, you will be ready to advocate for yourself in a positive and productive manner. It is better to make the best of it than quit and not graduate with the rest of your class. Never underestimate independent action as a great educator.

the best made plans will more than likely change before the day is over.

What can you do to make this successful? Good organizational skills are what you need to develop. At this point, your notebook should be organized so you can easily find what you need. The evening before, you will want to plan the next day as if it will go perfectly. Planning will save you from staying late to complete notes and treatments. The next element is small, frequent communications with your fieldwork educator. Every morning, check in with your fieldwork educator for a last-minute update for changes, such as new admissions, discharges, and cancellations. Check in again at lunchtime so you can juggle cases and adjust meeting times. At the end of your day, you should be able to see your day schedule completely checked off. Make notes for the next day, and remember that frequent communications will save you from

disaster. A somewhat more vague element that will help you is your attitude about change. This is a time to go with the flow, not expect perfection, and smile all the time. At times (see *How Should You Respond— Building or Burning Your Bridges?*), fieldwork might not go as well as expected, and being responsive to changes and adjustments may affect your future job prospects.

You might ask yourself, "Why am I doing all my fieldwork educator's work?" For the fieldwork educator to validate that you are "entry-level competent," you need to be able to handle a nearly full caseload. You might be competent to treat the many different types of cases before this stage, but it is a real test of your ability to be considered ready for independent job performance if you can perform at this level for at least a full week if not two.

Saying goodbye for many students is an emotionally laden learning experience. With your fieldwork educator, plan the best way to say goodbye to each client you are treating 2 weeks before you leave. It will not be the same for each client, as some will have difficulty seeing you leave. For those with cognitive deficits, frequent reminders help. This is another good time to write your feelings in a journal and share them with your fieldwork educator. Now that you are at the end, your notebook and journal are your remembrance and chronological summary of your learning experiences.

As you go through this stage, you will notice a subtle change in yourself. You will realize that with all the previous learning experiences, you have now developed your own style as a therapist or assistant. You will still admire your fieldwork educator for his or her expertise, but you will recognize your own areas of competence, feel confident in what you are doing, and see yourself as a unique and contributing member of our profession.

In this chapter, the art of learning in a nonacademic setting was explored, showing both the opportunities and the pitfalls that present themselves at each stage of fieldwork. Being aware of how you, the student, shape your own educational destiny by every word and action is key to your success. Choosing, reflecting, and deciding are techniques that the student perfects in fieldwork to be optimally ready for the real world of work.

REFERENCES

Cook, A. M., & Hussey, S. M. (1995). *Assistive technologies: Principles and practice.* St. Louis, MO: Mosby.

Crist, P. (1997). How students "Hit Fieldwork Running." *Advance for Occupational Therapists, 13,* 4.

Hall, N. (2001). *Winning the stress challenge.* Temple Terrace, FL: Institute for Health and Human Performance.

Johnson, S. (1998). *Who moved my cheese?* New York, NY: Putnam.

Section III

SUPERVISION

Chapter 9

TEAMS AND TEAMWORK

Donna Latella, MA, OTR

As a fieldwork student, you will become an integral part of a team, probably sooner than you anticipate. Particularly on level II fieldwork, your observations, interventions, objectivity, and "new vision" will be welcomed. This welcoming may not occur immediately or on its own. In many settings, particularly emerging practice areas where OT is new to the team, you may have to work on being accepted as a member. In searching the literature, there is a vast array of writing on teams and teamwork, although very little that incorporates students. This chapter will attempt to address fieldwork students as members of a team. By the end of the chapter, you will attempt the following objectives:

➡ Define a team.

➡ Explain the benefits and purpose of working on a team.

➡ Acknowledge practice areas where teams may work.

➡ Acknowledge three team approaches.

➡ Explain the roles of team members in emerging practice areas.

➡ Discuss skills for effective teamwork, collaboration, and communication.

➡ Acknowledge how fieldwork students become part of the team.

➡ Be prepared to report on a team and use supervision time to analyze performance.

WHAT IS A TEAM?

A team is a group of two or more individuals working together toward the achievement of specific goals. The health care team professionals represent different disciplines and share common values, while working toward common objectives. The team has a specific coordination of activity and operations amongst its members, and each group determines the rules of behavior and work. It is important for the team to perform its work as a single unit, allowing decisions to be made by consensus and good communication. The unit's main goal should be the welfare of the client over any other interests. With this in mind, the task of the team must be well understood and accepted by all members in order to achieve commitment and loyalty. Members should be free, however, to express their feelings and ideas, while understanding that conflict and disagreement are normal and necessary parts of the development of the team. Remember that a new team does not immediately become effective. Instead, it is developed through a process of consistent efforts and dedication of the leader and members.

BENEFITS OF TEAMS

As an occupational therapy student, there are many benefits when working on a health care team. Foremost, as a team member and student, you are finally able to put theory to practice by assimilating all of your clinical and professional skills into one package. You have learned about various other health care professions, and now you will see them in action. Most of all, you will observe others as role models in order to develop yourself as a team member. By observing others, you may tease out the negative characteristics observed and adopt the positive characteristics that most suit your personality. In the efforts to maximize your strengths as a clinician, you will find the team to be a means of support and growth. As a team member, you will learn invaluable lessons on becoming a leader and advocate for your clients and their families.

THE FIVE PS IN TEAM

Holpp (1999) introduces the five Ps—purpose, place, power, plan, and people—as a basic way to understand teams and their organization. These are discussed next.

Purpose

Purpose addresses the need to bring people together to collaborate, develop direction, develop commitment, and work interdependently. Health care teams, in particular, have the general purpose of client-focused care, which is holistic in nature and of high quality and efficiency. Specifically, a team should have a "vision," a sense of purpose or expectations for achievement. This vision should reflect the larger organization's mission statement, strategic plan, and goals. Holpp (1999) states that this purpose is a sense of what the team is expected to achieve within the context of the organizational vision. Of course, a team's vision will vary depending upon the clientele, setting, and team members.

Place

Place addresses the question how a team model fits into the organizational structure of a workplace or program. For example, are there typical or emerging practice areas that do not have a team model in place? Will a team model fit into many emerging practice arenas? Consider practice areas such as wellness and health promotion, independent living centers, homeless shelters, and day care centers. It is important to note that a team model does not fit into every health care setting or practice area. The needs of the clients and practitioners involved must be assessed when considering a team approach.

Power

Power addresses who takes the leadership or responsibilities of the team and the scope of work involved. Leadership may be passed from one member to another, depending upon the needs of the client and the approach (see Transdisciplinary Approach on p. 97). Leadership may be dictated by the type of setting in which the team occurs. For example, in a medical model, the team leader may be a physician, such as a psychiatrist or medical director. In a community model, the team leader may be a social worker or case manager. The leader is responsible for setting the agenda, inviting consultants as needed, delegating responsibilities, ensuring that the meeting runs accordingly, setting time limits, and providing follow-ups as needed.

Plan

Plan refers to the structure of the team and who will take on which responsibilities. Team approaches are part of the plan, as well. Optimal patient care and recovery are facilitated by the team effort of various disciplines combining their approaches. Specifically, a team will be organized and run according to one of three approaches in attempts to provide comprehensive, holistic, and optimal client-centered care. The three team approaches are as follows:

⟶ Multidisciplinary approach: Within this model, various disciplines work together where each professional has separate and distinctive roles. Assessment reports, recommendations, goals, and intervention strategies are also discipline-specific. Communication to other team members is either direct or indirect; thus, collaboration and coordination are not typically part of this approach. This approach tends to be expensive and less efficient with most clients. For example, an occupational therapy assistant may be working with a home care client on increasing independence in activities of daily living (ADLs) three mornings per week, while a certified nursing assistant (CNA) may provide morning care on the remaining days, unaware of the client's abilities, progress, and functional level.

⟶ Interdisciplinary approach: This model refers to disciplines working together on overlapping goals, allowing for an increased coordination of services. Team members collaborate on reports of assessments, goals, and intervention plans. Practitioners may also perform coassessments or interventions and share goals. Dunn (2000) states that team members negotiate priorities, and the intervention plan is a consensus of the group. An example of an interdisciplinary approach in an adult day care center might include an intervention shared by the OT and the art therapist as follows: The intervention is a watercolor painting activity. The OT's goal is for the client to independently hold a medium-sized brush successfully while painting. The art therapist's goal is for the client to explore his or her feelings behind the theme of the painting. Both therapists will collaborate their findings and recommendations with this model.

⟶ Transdisciplinary approach: This model involves all team members in cross training or "blurring" of roles by relinquishing predetermined boundaries. It maximizes the strength of the team members by requiring much flexibility and less duplication of services. Each discipline contributes information to the team process. Depending upon the specific needs of the client, one practitioner will then implement the intervention and become the team leader. For example, for a client who has family and financial issues impeding a realistic return to independent living, the team leader chosen might be the social worker. This individual would receive information and recommendations from other team members and would be responsible for contacting possible alternate living situations for the team to discuss. This approach is complicated and may be uncomfortable for students, as it requires members of the team to be experienced, flexible, and committed to the model.

People

Members truly make the team. Specific members vary depending on the needs of the clientele, the service provider, and whether discharge planning is required. The average team size is five members, with one being the team leader. Team members may be permanent or consultative in nature. For example, in a mental health setting, a physical therapist is probably not needed as a permanent team member, but may be called in as a consultant when a client requires a specific referral (see *Examples of Team Members* on p. 98).

Now that you know the five Ps, it is time to look at the details of your present team.

Student Activity 1

Fill in the following information to analyze the specifics of the team, for each of your affiliations, as appropriate.

⟶ Practice area.

⟶ Practice setting.

⟶ Title of team leader.

⟶ List team members and their roles.

⟶ Identify the team approach followed and explain reasoning.

⟶ Emerging practice areas may or may not use a team approach. It is important to analyze the service in order to determine if a team approach is applicable.

Student Activity 2

Consider emerging practice areas within the following exercise.

⟶ List at least three emerging practice areas.

⟶ Discuss why a team approach may or may not fit into this area.

⟶ List and discuss potential team members who may practice in this area, as appropriate.

EXAMPLES OF TEAM MEMBERS

- ➡ Physician/Psychiatrist
- ➡ Physician Specialist
- ➡ Physician Assistant
- ➡ Nurse/Nurse Practitioner or Specialist
- ➡ Certified Nursing Assistant
- ➡ Social Worker
- ➡ Occupational Therapist/Certified Occupational Therapy Assistant
- ➡ Physical Therapist/Physical Therapy Assistant
- ➡ Speech Therapist
- ➡ Recreation Therapist
- ➡ Dance Therapist
- ➡ Art Therapist

- ➡ Respiratory Therapist
- ➡ Dietician
- ➡ Teacher/Teacher's Aide
- ➡ Psychiatrist/Psychologist
- ➡ Chaplain
- ➡ Prosthetist/Orthotist
- ➡ Home Health Aide
- ➡ Dentist
- ➡ Pharmacist
- ➡ Exercise Physiologist
- ➡ Athletic Trainer
- ➡ Counselors
- ➡ Client/Family (to be decided by the team)

➡ Discuss the role of the occupational therapy practitioner within the emerging practice area team.

DYNAMICS OF TEAM DEVELOPMENT

Teams go through cycles of development gradually, allowing them to be capable of self-management. This is especially true as team members change, students join, or organization rules are modified. It is important for students and team members to understand this development in order to be prepared for the challenges a team may face. Holpp (1999), working off earlier writing of Tuckerman's study of group process, refers to the following four-phase model explaining how teams work:

- ➡ Forming—This phase is considered the "honeymoon" because it is filled with excitement, anxiety, and a feeling of power. Team members are getting familiar with each other before risks are taken, and the team is not very productive.

- ➡ Storming—This is the "posthoneymoon" phase where egos clash, personality differences surface, differences of opinion are obvious, and frustration increases. In this phase, new directions are suggested and evaluated, plans are made and revised, and ideas are proposed and challenged.

- ➡ Norming—This is the phase where "reality hits" because norms gradually develop and members get to know and understand each other. Productivity improves as the team forms a routine. The team's strengths and weaknesses are evident in this phase.

- ➡ Performing—This is the "synergy" phase because the team develops and grows. Relationships become clear, and a consensus regarding the team's direction is established. Goals are task-oriented, and the team is most productive.

Students should especially be aware of the phases of team development for a few important reasons. First of all, as a student, you will be entering into the team at any point in this development, and you should be prepared. An understanding of the team's developmental phase will help with your level of confidence, comfort, communication, and general ability to fit in. Second, anyone entering a team at any phase may disrupt the progress of the development. Even though you are a temporary addition to the team, the members must adjust to a student member. This team adjustment may be an extra challenge to members, causing feelings of frustration or anxiety. Your supervisor will help you with this adjustment and will likely be appreciative that you are aware of these development phases. Watching the changes a team goes through may be subtle or very obvious. In your journal, write down your daily observations and thoughts regarding these dynamics. Adding this information to your journal will help with the next activity.

SKILLS FOR EFFECTIVE TEAMWORK

- Knowledge of team member roles
- Knowledge of boundaries
- Knowledge of group process
- Good communication
- Empathy
- Collaboration
- Adherence to group rules
- Ability to respect others
- Ability to work in a group effort
- Self-awareness and self-confidence
- Flexibility
- Ability to problem solve

- Holistic thinking
- Productive use of supervision, feedback, and constructive criticism
- Assume responsibility
- Show team spirit
- Exude a positive attitude
- Appreciate differences in others
- Trust others
- Ability to handle conflict
- An open mind
- Commitment

Adapted from Latella, D. (2000). Teamwork in rehabilitation. In S Kumar (Ed.), *Multidisciplinary approach to rehabilitation* (pp. 27-42). Boston, MA: Butterworth Heinemann.

Student Activity 3

List and discuss the following regarding the team phase of development for each affiliation:

- Name and explain the phase of development that you feel the team is in at 2 weeks, at midterm, and in the final week of the affiliation. Discuss any changes you have observed.

- Discuss whether or not your participation as a team member has affected team development, communication, or progress. Are there positives and negatives? Give examples.

- Have other team members/students or your supervisor noted any change?

BECOMING A TEAM MEMBER

As an occupational therapy fieldwork student, becoming a member of the team may be a challenging process. It is especially challenging as the team acknowledges that a student is only a temporary member. As a new team member, you must work to earn the respect, trust, and acceptance of the established team. Before entering the team, it is important to establish which team approach is followed. Reviewing the previous section on team approaches before you begin fieldwork might be helpful. You must also learn the group's goals, process, policies, procedures, and rules. The roles, responsibilities, and leadership styles of each member are also important to observe. These considerations will assist you in the process of gradually fitting into the team (Latella, 2000).

Developing Teamwork Skills

Skills for Effective Teamwork

As a student, you most likely have had many opportunities during your education to practice teamwork skills, especially in group work. Beginning your affiliation, it is not expected that you will be an expert team member, but you should be ready to exemplify professionalism and a willingness to work on these skills. At the same time, you should realize your limitations and areas of growth to be cultivated while on affiliation. It is also important to learn from, and reflect upon, your experiences that occur within the framework of the team (see *Skills for Effective Teamwork*).

Collaboration and Communication

Students often have problems with collaboration and communication on fieldwork. As these are important and effective teamwork skills, they are addressed in more detail.

As a fieldwork student, you will be collaborating not only with professionals who are already established on a team but also with other students from the same or different disciplines who may also be members. For communication and collaboration to occur, each team member must have mutual respect for the expertise of the other. Collaboration is said to occur when diverse professionals share information, assessments, goals, and interventions regarding the same client. It also includes merging the expertise and perspectives of professionals with different backgrounds, dividing work according to expertise and interests, shifting leadership, and sharing ideas and support amongst team members (Lewis et al., 1998).

Collaboration also involves the coordination of efforts to achieve common goals and services provided to the client. This coordination requires regular team meetings in order for communication to occur and team relationships to develop. Team process is also involved with collaboration through the dynamics of team meetings. The dynamics are vital in allowing team members to have a comfort level for full participation, support, and trust.

Within team dynamics, good communication is essential. Good communication allows for free and open discussion, as well as efficient passing of information between members. Communication may not always be through a face-to-face team meeting. Communication may take the form of a phone call, documentation, or e-mail. Of course, face-to-face contact is most effective and allows for the best client confidentiality. Unfortunately, how team members communicate with each other is a major source of conflict in teams (Holpp, 1999).

Tips for good team communication include the following:

⟶ Ask open questions.

⟶ Practice active listening.

⟶ Deal directly and professionally with conflict and confrontation.

⟶ Periodically assess your own team spirit.

⟶ Create your own norm for politeness and respect.

⟶ Seek peer feedback.

THE TEAM MEETING—PREPARE

Consider your first team meeting, regardless of the affiliation setting or members involved. As a student, your first inclination may be to sit outside of the established team as a comfort-level notion. Instead, consider introducing yourself (or your supervisor may want to introduce you) at the start of the meeting and sitting within the circle of the team. Take this opportunity to listen and observe, not only in learning about the team members, but clients as well. It is recommended to take notes during the meeting. This will assist in your remembering the names and roles of each member and the details about clients. Also, write down any questions that you may need to ask your supervisor after the meeting.

Before the next team meeting, keep running notes about clients and issues that you have observed, and use strategies that may help you to remember names of team members. Talk with your supervisor regarding when he or she may want you to begin reporting on clients you are following. Use time outside of the fieldwork setting to review textbook information about diagnoses, interventions, and any other pertinent issues. Prepare educated questions to ask your supervisor. Your preparation will assist you in the event that a team member asks you a question about a client you are following, even before you formally report.

THE TEAM MEETING—REPORT

After having observed a few team meetings, your supervisor will most likely ask you to report on client(s) you are following. It is important to exude as much confidence as possible. With this in mind, here are a few tips:

⟶ Refer to "tips for good team communication."

⟶ Meet with your supervisor, and ask questions/advice prior to reporting.

⟶ Take notes, which can be referred to when reporting.

⟶ Assume an "open" posture.

⟶ Maintain eye contact with all team members.

⟶ Speak in a volume loud enough for everyone to hear and with confidence.

⟶ Consider others' opinions/comments and dialogue with them.

Analyzing Performance Through Supervision

Supervision times are a great format for analyzing your contribution to the team and for using feedback constructively. During supervision meetings, it is suggested to ask your supervisor not only for constructive feedback on your performance during the team meeting, but also to possibly role-play more effective reporting styles or communication with other team members. Remember to use this feedback in a manner in which it can be fit into your communication style and personality. It is also important for you to self-analyze your performance and communication style. This can be done through journaling or keeping the meeting notes you have used to report from. Collaborating and role-playing with other students are other excellent means of providing feedback. The following activity provides a means of charting your progress as a team member during each week of affiliation. Remember to use your self-reflection as well as the feedback given by others.

Student Activity 4

Analyze your teamwork skills on a weekly basis while on each affiliation.

➡ Name:

➡ Site:

➡ Week #:

➡ Synopsis of your report in team meeting:

➡ Synopsis of team efforts/collaboration or communications outside of team meeting:

➡ Strengths noted:

➡ Weaknesses noted:

➡ Feedback from supervisor/others:

➡ Improvements made/skills achieved:

➡ Goals for improvement:

CONCLUSION

This chapter has attempted to introduce you to the basics regarding teamwork, particularly as an affiliating student. However, much of your learning will actually occur on the job, and it is dependent upon the setting, practice area, and supervision involved. Again, becoming a valued team member is a process that may take much time, even possibly well beyond your affiliations and into the first job. This process will involve learning from your mistakes as well as from the example of others. Remember to use your supervisory times well and use feedback, as appropriate. Your growth toward successful communication and collaboration is key to successful client-centered care. Always remember that, whether you are an affiliating student or an employee, you are an important member of the team with invaluable contributions.

REFERENCES

Dunn, W. (2000). *Best practice occupational therapy: In community service with children and families.* Thorofare, NJ: SLACK Incorporated.

Holpp, L. (1999). *Managing teams.* New York, NY: McGraw Hill Co., Inc.

Latella, D. (2000). Teamwork in rehabilitation. In S. Kumar (Ed.), *Multidisciplinary approach to rehabilitation.* Boston, MA: Butterworth Heinemann.

Lewis, R., Tucker, R., Tsao, H., Canaan, E., Bryant, J., Talbot, P., et al. (1998). Improving interdisciplinary team process: A practical approach to team development. *J Allied Health, 27*(2), 89-95.

SUGGESTED READINGS

American Occupational Therapy Association. (1996). *The occupational therapy manager* (revised ed.). Bethesda, MD: Author.

Castledine, G. (1996). Encouraging team collaboration in healthcare. *British Journal of Nursing, 5,* 14.

Fordyce, W. (1981). On interdisciplinary peers. *Arch Phys Med Rehabil, 62,* 51-53.

Heruti, R., & Ohry, A. (1995). The rehabilitation team: A commentary. *Am J Phys Med Rehabil, 74,* 466-468.

Jelles, F., van Bennekom, C., & Lankhurst, G. (1995). The interdisciplinary team conference in rehabilitation medicine, a commentary. *Am J Phys Med Rehabil, 74,* 464-465.

Katzenbach, J., & Smith, D. (1999). *The wisdom of teams.* New York, NY: McKinsey & Company, Inc.

Kouzes, J. M., & Posner, B. Z. (1987). *The leadership challenge: How to get extraordinary things done in organizations.* San Francisco, CA: Jossey-Bass.

Keith, R. A. (1991). The comprehensive treatment team in rehabilitation. *Arch Phys Med Rehabil, 72,* 269-274.

Ling, C. (1996). Performance of a self-directed work team in a home health care agency. *J Nurs Adm, 26,* 36-40.

McKeehan, K. (1981). *Continuing care: A multidisciplinary approach to discharge planning.* St. Louis, MO: Mosby.

Mears, P. (1994). *Health care teams.* Delray Beach, FL: St. Lucie Press.

Mullins, L., Balderson, B., Sanders, N., Chaney, J., & Whatley, P. (1997). Therapists' perceptions of team functioning in rehabilitation contexts. *International Journal of Rehabilitation and Health, 3*(4), 281-288.

Purtillo, R. (1988). Ethical issues in teamwork: The context of rehabilitation. *Arch Phys Med Rehabil, 69,* 318-322.

Purtillo, R., & Haddad, A. (1996). *Health professional and patient interaction* (5th ed.). Philadelphia, PA: W. B. Saunders, Co.

Sladyk, K. (1997). *OT student primer: A guide to college success.* Thorofare, NJ: SLACK Incorporated.

Chapter 10

SUPERVISION

Mary Alicia Barnes, OTR
Amy Lynne Thornton, MS, OTR

The supervisory relationship holds tremendous potential and is a key component to achieving success in your occupational therapy (OT) career. As you enter into this interactive relationship, it is important to understand what supervision is, what it is not, and your role throughout the process. As with any relationship, the supervisory one can be complex. There are principles and practices of supervision that can build your knowledge and skills to help you effectively engage in the supervisory relationship and process. Your ability to learn the crucial interpersonal skills involved in the process of supervision will ultimately determine your ability to be successful and will aid in the achievement of your full potential. As a supervisee, you, your clients, and your practice will benefit if you understand your roles and responsibilities in the mutual learning process that supervision can provide. This chapter will guide you in learning about the dynamic roles and relationships of supervisor and supervisee throughout your course of professional development. This chapter will do the following:

➡ Discuss fundamentals that contribute to successful supervisory relationships.

➡ Share tips for getting started.

➡ Provide a few journal exercises designed to help you prepare for entering new systems and starting new relationships.

➡ Highlight components of the supervisory relationship, such as communication styles and various tasks and roles of supervisor and supervisee.

➡ Identify some factors that contribute to successful performance as well as a few pitfalls to avoid.

During your OT career, you will experience many different types of supervision. In some instances, other professionals or an individual who is unfamiliar with OT may provide supervision. You may have more than one supervisor, and supervision may occur in one-to-one or group formats. Models of supervision can be collaborative (one supervisor to two or more students), can involve multiple mentors (two supervisors to one or more students), or be a hybrid of these models (two supervisors to two or more students) (Barnes & Evenson, 2000). Each model provides unique benefits and possible challenges that emerge from the different relationships they require.

Providing supervision and making good use of supervision are skills that take time to learn and develop with practice. Individuals vary in their styles and approaches to the supervisory relationship; you should not expect any two supervisors or your relationship with them to be the same. Each supervision opportunity should be viewed as a new relationship that builds upon previous knowledge and experience. With each new beginning, look carefully at your expectations of yourself and others as you engage in the supervisory relationship.

BUILDING THE SUPERVISORY FOUNDATION

Initial contact with your prospective supervisor is an important step in establishing your relationship. This may be a phone conversation, a voice mail, an e-mail or mail correspondence, an informal meeting, or a formally arranged interview. First impressions can be significant, and it is important that you represent yourself well. Being open and honest is a crucial step toward building trust in your working alliance with your supervisor. Prior to your initial contact, you may want to consider what it is you bring to the situation and supervisory relationship.

For your initial meeting with your supervisor you may want to bring the following:

➡ A calendar or a date book planner.

➡ A résumé tailored to the practice setting or experience.

➡ A brief written summary of your learning and communication style.

➡ An outline of interests you hope to explore or goals you hope to achieve during the experience.

➡ A set of questions about subjects such as theories used in the setting, intervention outcome measures, or research/evidence-based practice initiatives.

In addition, asking for written materials about the setting or program, such as information about the philosophy and codes of conduct, might be a way to begin learning about the setting. You might also inquire about recommended resources or reading suggestions to study. Taking steps to learn about the setting and systems can assist you in your preparation for fieldwork experiences and your relationship with your supervisor.

Student Activity

As you enter a new setting or practice situation, it is important to take time to prepare. The following questions are designed to act as a semistructured journal. This activity aims to be an exercise in self-discovery regarding your thoughts and feelings as you enter into fieldwork experiences. We recommend that you revise this activity each time you encounter a new experience. This activity format can serve as a means of preparing yourself and monitoring each phase of your professional development.

Bearing in mind the context of your upcoming fieldwork placement, briefly record your answers to the following questions:

➡ What do I see as the definition of OT?

➡ How comfortable am I in sharing my definition and explaining OT to others?

➡ How do I envision OT benefiting this setting and the population served?

➡ How would I tailor my definition of OT to fit this setting?

➡ What do I see as my strengths in this particular environment or practice arena?

➡ What are my hopes for this particular learning experience or opportunity?

➡ What are my fears about this upcoming experience?

➡ What are my areas for growth?

➡ What personal biases might I bring? Give an example.

Review what you have recorded. After reviewing your responses, answer the following questions:

➡ Are you able to articulate your definition of OT and to modify it in addressing those with whom you will work?

➡ In what way might your perceptions about OT or what is to be learned be a form of bias?

➡ What other biases might you have based upon your own experience/cultural identity?

Often, when entering into a new supervisory relationship, the supervisor may also have hopes and fears about the experience or biases, whether they are conscious or unconscious. Acknowledging your own hopes, fears, and biases can be a first step toward being open-minded. Realizing and accepting differences can help you to identify ways in which you can grow personally and professionally. Each fieldwork opportunity and supervisory relationship can offer a means for you to increase your understanding of yourself and others.

The following account highlights the importance of taking the time to reflect on and be aware of some of the issues addressed by the previous journal exercise.

Personal Narrative: Timing is Many Things

An opportunity to work with adolescent boys in a juvenile justice facility seemed like an exciting summer project that would allow us to explore opportunities for integrating OT into a nontraditional setting. In our haste to begin, we went to the facility and presented our ideas about running an art group for the boys to the director, who was our site supervisor, but not an occupational therapist.

Our 8-week group series became riddled with administrative and systems issues, such as being locked out of the facility due to security system malfunctions, not having our meeting space ready, not having the agreed upon members for the group, and poor communication with the director (our supervisor), as well as agency staff and clinicians. Even though we had scheduled appointments to discuss our work, our supervisor was often unavailable for meetings, and when we did meet, our supervisor seemed distracted and somewhat detached from our group program agenda. We felt frustrated, somewhat discouraged, and at times questioned our direction and purpose in working with this agency.

Off-site OT supervision, facilitated by our fieldwork coordinator, was held back at our academic program. These supervision sessions became a time to explore and share our feelings about our experience. Through this exchange, we were able to step back from the situation and regain perspective about what, in fact, we were learning and doing. We shared our reactions and discussed how our initial expectations were much different from the actual outcome. We ascertained

that, despite the fact that things did not turn out as we had initially expected, we were learning about the boys, their needs, system issues, as well as our own strengths and challenges as group leaders, including how to use our skills in building therapeutic relationships. We gathered written feedback from the boys, who indicated that our groups provided them with a means for sharing their feelings and managing their stress.

In retrospect, we realized that this opportunity provided a valuable lesson about the importance of taking the time to understand what a system's and supervisor's needs and expectations are before identifying how we as occupational therapy students can best be of service and attempt to address these needs. We learned that we should have done a literature search and self-directed readings to increase our knowledge about the population and system that we had endeavored to serve. We discovered that we were overly eager to meet our own agenda of providing a group structure before the system was really ready. We were able to acknowledge that we chose our plan because it seemed like the most obvious need and a convenient plan at the time. We were able to accept that, in reality, our plan was based on what we felt comfortable doing, what we knew had been done before at this agency, the 8-week time frame we had, and what little we knew about the juvenile justice system. At the end of the experience, when we shared some of our reflections with our site supervisor, he revealed to us that he had indeed been preoccupied with major systems issues around security, program overhaul, and staff turnover. He stated that he, too, had hoped to be more available and supportive. We all agreed that the experience, though not at all what we had expected, had still been a meaningful and worthwhile venture for ourselves and the population we served.

GETTING STARTED IN SUPERVISION

Getting familiar with a new situation, setting, roles, and people can be overwhelming. Learning the system and the players takes time and deserves your attention in order to optimally form collaborative relationships. The stresses of a new situation can be a challenging first step. Often, you can become overloaded with a tremendous amount of information. You may recognize yourself responding negatively to the stress in the form of experiencing tension, feeling lost or confused, or becoming withdrawn (Barnes & Evenson, 1997). This response is a natural part of your transition, and, as you become acclimated to the setting, it should diminish.

This reaction to a new situation is referred to as an "orientation response" (Toffler, as cited in Butler, 1972), which is your brain's and body's effort to adjust. This process can place "extra demands on the body's energy and cause significant changes in body chemistry" (p. 403), which can interfere with your ability to process the new material. As a result of the stress of feeling over-stimulated or overwhelmed, you may become less efficient and feel fatigued. You can try to minimize the effects of an "orientation response" by preparing for your initial entry into a new environment. One strategy that might be helpful is to have a notebook or system for recording:

➡ Questions

➡ Observations

➡ Reactions

➡ Tips regarding policies/protocols or other key information shared with you

➡ A "to do" list regarding tasks to perform or items to look up or review

➡ A method for organizing items such as your daily schedule and necessary forms or paperwork.

Another strategy that may help you prepare is to try to understand your own communication style. Understanding your communication style and the styles of the people you work with can increase the effectiveness of your communication. One popular method of exploring communication styles is through the use of formal inventories similar to those used to identify learning styles. One such tool, the Martin Operating Styles Inventory (Martin & Martin, 1989), clusters the characteristic approaches people use to communicate into four categories: thinker, feeler, sensor, and intuitor. These styles of communicating are briefly described below.

COMMUNICATION STYLES

Thinkers

Thinkers are logical and like just the facts. Thinkers are analytical and prefer an orderly process. They are interested in the purpose, standards, or significance applied to what is being discussed. Thinkers prefer a quiet, neat, and organized workspace.

Feelers

Feelers deduce information via their emotions. They value relationships and may make decisions based upon "what 'feels' right" (Martin & Martin, 1989).

Feelers like to use humor and try to establish a work climate that is friendly and harmonious.

Sensors

Sensors gather and filter information through the five senses. They respond quickly to what is happening around them and are very active, often multi-tasking. Their work environment is likely to be lively and cluttered.

Intuitors

Intuitors like to think about information from a big picture perspective. They often seem able to see possibilities that do not seem evident to others. They are imaginative, innovative, and like to take risks. Intuitors may seem preoccupied with their own thoughts, and projects or work yet to be finished may be all around their workspace (Martin & Martin, 1989).

Student Activity 1

Review the descriptions of communication styles listed above. Choose which one(s) seems to best describe you. Think about a situation where you felt that you were experiencing difficulty in communicating with someone about something that was important to you. Try to identify the communication style you feel best suits the person with whom you were trying to communicate. Rework the situation and try to communicate your point using an approach that is more compatible with the other person's communication style.

If communicating with a thinker, try using the following:

➡ The purpose behind…

➡ I think the following…

➡ The fact of the matter is…

➡ The significance would be…

If communicating with a feeler, try using the following:

➡ What I'm feeling about the situation is that we should…

➡ My gut reaction would be to…

➡ What seems best for all involved is to…

If communicating with a sensor, try

➡ What I'm hearing/seeing/sensing is…

➡ What I'd like to do is…

➡ The steps of my action plan would be to…

If communicating with an intuitor, try using the following:

➡ In general…

➡ I imagine that...

➡ I'd like to try...

➡ What I'm wondering is...

Prior to your fieldwork, it may be beneficial to prepare a brief summary about your communication style to share with your supervisor. Together, you might examine how your style coincides with your supervisor's style and expectations. Doing this may help you to assess if and when you will need to adapt your style to enhance the quality of your communication with others.

As with learning styles, we all use a combination of these communication approaches, but usually have one or two that are more prominent and therefore are used most often. It is the synergy that comes from a combination of all these styles that can make a working group most productive. Knowing your preferred communication style, having the ability to be flexible, and adapting your behavior as best you can to better correspond with others' communication styles can lead to more efficient and effective interactions.

BEGINNING THE SUPERVISORY PROCESS

When starting in a supervisory relationship, it is helpful to try to share your perceived needs and expectations. Having this exchange and clarifying what to expect from each other helps to define the parameters of the supervisory time as well as venues for learning. This discussion may also help prevent misunderstandings, confusion, and oversights. Discussing specific expectations such as your role during meetings or sessions with clients and when to ask questions or share reflections and setting a time for processing your thoughts and reactions can prevent lapses or miscommunication. Try to denote the best times and structures for these types of communication. For example, it may be informal verbal processing. This might be done briefly during or after sessions or in a daily morning or afternoon check in. The processing might take the form of a more formal verbal or written report, summarized during a weekly supervision time. There may be structured observation worksheets or log assignments for you to complete to guide your focus and enhance your learning (Barnes & Evenson, 2000) by linking your academic knowledge to the practice environment. These types of assignments also serve to provide your supervisor with more detailed information about your knowledge and ability level.

SUPERVISION: TASKS AND ROLES

The primary role of a supervisor is to maintain the provision of quality care for individuals receiving services while simultaneously facilitating learning. Supervisors, therefore, have an administrative and an evaluative role. They have a professional responsibility to uphold standards by which competency is measured. Often, they will do this by establishing behavioral objectives or minimum competencies that serve as a means to measure a supervisee's performance. In this way, a supervisee's progress toward demonstrating competency as an entry-level practitioner is monitored. Specific behavioral objectives or minimum competencies tailored to the setting are usually written to augment or complement the American Occupational Therapy Association, Inc. (AOTA) Fieldwork Evaluation Forms (AOTA, 1983, 1987), which frequently serve as the official documentation of a student's fieldwork performance.

Supervisors can function as a resource or subject expert, a guide, a potential role model, and a "sounding board" (Curtis, 1985). A supervisor can be an advisor, instructing you in specific material or techniques, or a collaborator, supporting and empowering you as you apply theory to practice. Ideally, a supervisor creates a learning atmosphere that is safe, motivating, and developmentally appropriate to you, the learner. A supervisor should not play the role of parent/guardian, friend, or your therapist (Crist, 1996). Staying aware of your interpersonal boundaries is important. Doing so can help you monitor yourself so you realize when you might be transferring characteristics of more familiar relationships into the supervisory relationship.

There is a delicate balance of power in the dynamics of the supervisory relationship. Successful outcomes require each person in the supervisory relationship to be aware of their roles and responsibilities and to actively engage in the learning process. Your supervisor's responsibility is to ensure you have met the required minimum standards or expectations for skilled entry-level role performance. Your responsibility is to take initiative and demonstrate enthusiasm as a learner. You need to develop the ability to think on your feet and demonstrate your comfort with the process of learning by reflecting your willingness to learn how to learn. You should convey your interest and investment in learning what you need to know. As an OT practitioner, you will need to be proactive, recognizing that the knowledge base of the profession is constantly growing and that change is always going to happen. Accepting this nature of the profession and striving to anticipate and respond to change is an important step in your professional journey. These are the skills and qualities that will be essential to your success in your chosen career of OT.

Sometimes, establishing the degree of supervisor versus supervisee control and defining your roles in the learning and supervisory process may be complicated. Time constraints, people's beliefs about their roles, and/or their experiences in other supervisory situations or roles (as a learner or supervisor) may make them uneasy with the process this negotiation involves. You may feel like the roles are somewhat unclear. Your supervisor's aim of trying to promote self-direction in you as the learner, while ensuring that specific learning outcomes are achieved, may seem paradoxical at times. This ambiguity may result in some discomfort on your part, which may emerge as you taking a rejecting stance or experiencing difficulty in adapting to your supervisor's approach. At different phases of the experience, you may struggle with wanting more control or feeling like you have been given too much responsibility in the learning process or supervisory relationship. Remember that, ultimately, while supervisors can assume varying degrees of influence in your learning process, the final outcome is really up to you. Finding ways to discuss with your supervisor your understanding of the distribution of power in the supervisory relationship and what it means for you may help you establish your roles within the relationship.

There will always be a role of authority for your supervisor in your supervisory relationship. This is to be expected, as your supervisor's role is to evaluate and monitor your performance. This does not mean that your supervisory relationship cannot be caring and reciprocal. Although you may express concern for one another, it is important to respect the boundaries and limits of the supervisory relationship in order for it to be most effective and objective. Interacting in a more companionable manner may ease the anxiety of a new relationship; however, it may lead to a disruption in the balance of the roles of supervisor and supervisee. You may find yourself struggling with issues of dependency or of autonomy, wanting your supervisor to be with you when he or she is not needed or wanting to be on your own before you are truly ready. Relating socially as a peer to your supervisor may also interfere with your ability to give and receive feedback or to disclose important information about what you are feeling or thinking regarding your fulfillment of your student role.

Student Activity 2

Exploring meaning and power balance in relationships is difficult. The following semistructured journal is designed to help you try to honestly reflect on your expectations of your supervisory relationship. Examining past relationships and experiences may provide insights as to what might be influencing you as you participate in your supervisory relationship.

➡ What are my past experiences of supervision?

➡ What am I looking for in a supervisor?

➡ Am I able to differentiate what I want versus what I need for supervision?

➡ What do I bring to this relationship?

➡ Am I aware of the differences between what I look for in a friend versus a supervisor?

➡ What is my level of comfort with having my performance evaluated and receiving feedback?

➡ What is my level of comfort with giving feedback?

➡ What is the minimum amount and means of contact I feel would adequately facilitate my learning (per day? per week? in person? by phone or e-mail?)?

➡ Am I ready to be self-directed or assume responsibility for my own learning?

What are some examples of how I would/could go about this? Often, a simple cause of tension in a supervisory relationship is differing expectations. In reviewing your responses, ask yourself the following question: Do my expectations seem reasonable or realistic?

If so, briefly summarize your responses in a manner you feel you could relay them to a potential supervisor. If not, where can you adjust your expectations?

After each supervisory experience, review and revise your responses as you prepare for the next step of your professional journey.

AIMING FOR SUCCESS

Supervisors and students (Herzberg, 1994; Tinson, 1999) have identified what they consider the characteristics of successful fieldwork students. Both groups identified flexibility and teamwork as extremely important. Other skills seen as noteworthy included time management, effective communication, and problem solving. Students also identified honesty, professionalism, and good judgment as contributing factors in their success (Tinson, 1999). Being proactive or self-directed as well as willing to actively experiment and learn by doing were attributes in students clearly valued by supervisors (Herzberg, 1994).

Student Activity 3

Use the scale below (adapted from Herzberg, 1994; Tinson, 1999) to evaluate yourself according to the list of characteristics attributed to successful fieldwork students.

Rate yourself on a scale of 1-5: At this stage of my OT education, I...

1 = have or can demonstrate this skill/characteristic

2 = am developing this skill/characteristic

3 = am developing a plan to improve this skill/characteristic

4 = am aware that I need to develop this skill/characteristic but have no plan

5 = have no idea about myself in relation to this skill/characteristic

___ flexibility
___ teamwork
___ time management
___ communication
___ problem solving
___ honesty
___ professionalism
___ good judgment
___ self-direction
___ a willingness to actively experiment and learn by doing

If you received a total score of more than 30, you might want to consider seeking advice and input from someone, such as an academic advisor, faculty member, or fieldwork coordinator. Ask this person if he or she can be of help to you in developing a learning contract or plan to assist you in developing the necessary skills/characteristics to support your being successful.

The task of knowing yourself is a daunting one. Just when you think you know who you are and what you want, your life may change, you may surprise yourself and change your mind, or you may begin to question what it is that you really want or need. When entering a supervisory relationship, it is helpful to share things about yourself, such as your perceived learning style and what you see as your strengths and challenges as a learner. Relating what you understand at present about your personality may also be useful. A part of who you are is how you respond to stressful situations. Fieldwork is often a time of transition, and you may

experience varying amounts of stress as your identity as an OT practitioner develops. Some of the stress you will experience is useful—it keeps you attentive and can be energizing when channeled toward being productive. An excessive amount of stress can impede your performance and negatively affect your well-being. Understanding your tolerance for stress and your process for dealing with it is a vital component of successful fieldwork. You will need to explore and identify ways of adapting to and coping with stress.

Healthy ways of coping involve seeking support and taking action in ways that are problem-focused and solution-oriented (Mitchell & Kampfe, 1990). Signs that you are not coping well include becoming avoidant, using escapism, and having distorted thought patterns such as denial, "wishful thinking," and/or blaming yourself (Mitchell & Kampfe, 1990). Distorted thinking often falls into three patterns: absolutist, catastrophizing, and shoulds (Curtis, 1985). Absolutist thinking, characterized by an "all or nothing" attitude or belief, occurs when your view of things becomes inflexibly concrete, commonly referred to as "black or white" thinking. You believe things must either be wrong or right, with no middle ground. Catastrophizing is a distorted thought process which takes the most pessimistic view possible, blowing events out of proportion. Shoulds are when you begin to make extreme generalizations about the way things "should" be or the way others "should" behave, which results in your imposing unattainable standards on yourself or others.

These types of thought processes may be based on beliefs you hold about yourself or expectations that stem from idealism rather than realism. These ways of thinking are irrational and may surface when you are faced with a stressful situation. Distorted thinking can occur as part of an emotional reaction to events, when you feel overwhelmed and lose your perspective. It can add to your stress level and have a negative effect, not only on your performance, but on your relationships with others as well.

Understanding the interplay of the elements of your personality, learning style, and mechanisms of coping may help you to predict how you will respond to the social and situational contexts of learning on fieldwork. Investing time in self-assessment and self-reflection about your personality, your strengths and challenges as a learner, and how you respond to and cope with stress can allow you to do the following:

1. Anticipate potential areas of difficulty.

2. Identify growth needs.

3. Distinguish where you may need support and assistance.

Communicating openly and honestly about yourself may help you create a framework for your supervision built on realistic expectations and respect for you as an individual and your learning needs. Through this process, you can sort out what might be useful to address in supervision in relation to your performance in the practice context.

Supervision: Process and Context

Despite our possible preconceptions of it as a concrete action, supervision is a very dynamic and abstract notion. As you, the supervisee, change and grow, your supervisor's actions are likely to shift. A supervisory approach may also be contextual or dependent upon the situation. For example, the structure and format may vary during level I fieldwork experiences, which are designed to increase your "comfort level with and understanding of the needs of clients" (Accreditation Council for Occupational Therapy Education [ACOTE], 1998a, 1998b) and to provide you with exposure to "various aspects of the OT process" (ACOTE, 1998a, 1998b). Level I fieldwork may occur in a 4-hour site visit or through observation made several days during the course of a week. There may be longer scheduling formats that allow for more of a participatory role. Visiting for a few hours a week extending over a time period of several months, or as an intensive 3-week experience prior to or at the end of a semester are some examples of these formats. In level I fieldwork, your supervisory relationship is usually not as intensely collaborative as it may be on level II fieldwork.

Level II fieldwork has more defined standards and is a National Board for Certification in Occupational Therapy (NBCOT) requirement. Level II fieldwork can encompass up to 960 hours of training, depending on your level of training degree (occupational therapist versus OT assistant), and is typically done in two fieldwork placements. The goal of level II fieldwork is to promote clinical reasoning, reflective practice, and competent entry-level practitioners (ACOTE, 1998a, 1998b). These aims require a significant investment in the supervisory relationship to ensure successful outcomes.

Starting out in a supervisory relationship, you are generally unfamiliar with the tasks necessary to perform your OT practitioner role. You are lacking some of the necessary skills you are there to learn through experience. This is a period of transition for you from an academic or classroom approach to learning, which can often be passive, to a more active phase in which learning often occurs through experimentation, doing, and discovery (Tyrssenaar & Perkins, 2001).

The developmental process of supervision generally takes you through different stages or phases. Each phase is dependent on your needs and abilities as a supervisee and the resultant actions of the supervisor. The nature of the process may be cyclical, depending upon what you encounter and master in your learning situation. Your supervisor may adopt a gradual approach that changes according to your development at each stage of the process. These stages are delineated below and are based on a four-stage model best described by referring to the supervisors' actions and role. These stages of supervision are called *directing*, *coaching*, *supporting*, and *delegating* (Ebb, McCoy, & Pugh, 1993). Below, we describe what typically occurs in each phase or stage of the supervisory process.

Directing

At this early phase in supervision, your supervisory relationship is just beginning, and you do not know each other yet. Your supervisor knows the tasks well and may provide you with a significant amount of direction. Your supervisor will most likely work closely with you at this point, and he or she may take responsibility for setting the structure of the day. This could involve orienting you to and engaging you in specific tasks chosen to evaluate your level of competency. Through these activities, your supervisor will determine your readiness to work directly with others (clients or other team members) or to assume specific roles (evaluation, intervention, documentation, group leadership) and the level of your involvement. It may be helpful at this point to try to map out your learning goals and a plan for achieving them over the time frame in which you will be in the setting. By doing this, you can establish a few clear progress markers and a relevant timeline in which to achieve them. Some supervisors have activities sketched out by a daily, weekly, or quarterly format that can serve as a template for this process.

This initial phase of your fieldwork and supervisory relationship can be a time of great expectations (Tyrssenaar & Perkins, 2001). Your confidence may be high, and you may be unaware of what it is you know or do not know. As you realize possible information gaps, it is your role and responsibility to identify and address when you are unfamiliar with a term, concept, theory base, or procedure. The mark of a competent professional is his or her ability to admit his or her knowledge deficit and actively take initiative to learn the material. This may involve using your own time to review academic material or gather resources or information. When realizing you may not know something, it is useful to wonder why that might be the case, but it is not helpful to take a defensive stance of blaming (your supervisor, your professors/academic program, or even yourself). You could consult with your supervisor for recommended courses of action (e.g., readings, talking with a subject matter expert, library or Internet search), network with your peers, or follow up with resource people from your academic institution. These types of activities are part of what it means to be engaged in life-long learning. It is important to be accountable for your own learning and to value the process.

Coaching

As you gain skill, becoming more proficient and competent in applying what you know and are learning, your supervisor may transition to serving more as a coach. Your relationship becomes focused on talking about your ideas and rationales for what you are doing. At this phase, you may feel less confident than you did originally as you become more aware of the realities of practice (Tyrssenaar & Perkins, 2001). Your supervisor always retains the ultimate responsibility in regard to client care. However, at this phase in your supervisory relationship, he or she may await your suggestions and then take an active role in the final decision making in regard to an evaluation or intervention method to be implemented. Due to time constraints and logistics, a level I fieldwork supervisory relationship may not have time to develop beyond this coaching phase.

With increased time, your supervisory relationship broadens as your supervisor gets to know you better. Most likely, he or she will continue to work actively with you to plan and structure what you are doing. As the supervisee, demonstrating your abilities to think critically, problem-solve, work independently, and take responsibility is crucial at this stage. You must articulate your thought processes in order to show your readiness and ability to adapt to your emerging role as entry-level practitioner (Barnes & Evenson, 2000).

One mode for demonstrating your critical thinking abilities is to give your supervisor written summaries regarding areas in which you feel limited and to list possible solutions or ideas for improving the situation. Another method is to come to supervision prepared with an agenda of what you would like to discuss. These strategies can help you effectively make use of your supervisory sessions. You can use a simple log format for this process that identifies the following:

➡ What went well this week?

➡ What was challenging?

➡ What strategies did I use to address the challenges?

➡ What are my goals for next week? (Sullivan, 1997).

As you continue your professional development, you should be able to self-assess your progress by reflecting on and monitoring your feelings, thoughts, and actions. The focus of your supervision should shift to helping you differentiate not only what it is you know, but how you will synthesize your knowledge and put your learning goals into action. Take initiative to explain your thought process to others, telling them what you are thinking, what you are planning, and why. This can mean talking with your supervisor, reporting to other professionals, and/or discussing with individuals with whom you are working and their families/significant others or caregivers what your OT services entail.

You need to be mindful of how you are feeling about your performance and to find ways to effectively and professionally communicate this to your supervisor during supervision. The end of this coaching stage in the supervisory relationship often coincides with the midpoint of your fieldwork experience. A midterm evaluation is usually conducted at this time during a level II fieldwork placement. During the midterm evaluation of your performance and progress, it is useful to review your learning goals and activities you may have mapped out during the initial phase of your supervisory relationship. As mentioned earlier in this chapter, the site may have written criteria by which they delineate expected performance of entry-level practitioners in their setting, often referred to as behavioral objectives for level II fieldwork. It may be helpful to review the targeted expectations at this time. This can help you to delineate your progress and outline areas for your goals to focus on in the next phase of your learning.

You should also discuss with your supervisor the parameters for this evaluative session. For example, in plotting the overall course for your fieldwork, is your midterm performance evaluation based on what is typically expected from a student at this point? Or, is the measure of your performance at the midpoint based on what is to be expected as a final outcome (i.e., the expectations of an entry-level practitioner at the facility)? Bearing the standard of measure in mind, you should complete your own self-assessment of your performance for the midterm evaluation. Comparing and contrasting your rating of your performance with your supervisor's will help you to gauge how you each view your performance, noting your strengths and areas in need of improvement. The consistency between your ratings will provide useful information about the accuracy of your self-assessment. If your ratings differ, that can be an opportunity to look at why this may be the case. If you rate yourself higher than your supervisor's ratings of your performance, this is an opportunity to review expectations. If you rate yourself lower than your supervisor did, this can be an opportunity to explore why you feel this way about your skills and, if applicable, to gain some validation.

At this stage in the supervisory process, you should demonstrate that you are capable of the following:

➟ Planning and setting your own schedule.

➟ Identifying priorities and goals for your work with clients.

➟ Expressing chosen methods or modalities to evaluate and/or address client problems, as appropriate to your professional role (occupational therapist versus OT assistant).

➟ Documenting your services with improved clarity, fluency, and organization.

➟ Recognizing areas in which additional information/learning is necessary.

➟ Seeking resources to address learning and growth needs (Barnes & Evenson, as cited in Crist & McCarron, 2000).

Supporting

As your skills, comfort, and confidence grow, your supervisor may play more of a supportive role. You will be expected to take on more responsibility and a lead role in providing client care. Certainly, there may be moments of self-doubt and concern about your competence (Tyrssenaar & Perkins, 2001). At this stage, supervision becomes more focused on providing assurance and support (Crist & McCarron, 2000). Your supervisor may step back, allowing you to function more independently. His or her role shifts to one of actively listening to facilitate your problem solving and decision making (Curtis, 1985). You and your supervisor start to relate less about specific tasks and more about your overall performance.

This phase of the supervisory relationship becomes a time for you to look for opportunities to explore issues of your practice in greater depth. You can also use your supervisor as a sounding board to test some of your assumptions about how you are doing, some hypotheses about client issues and needs, and how prepared you are to function in the capacity of entry-level practitioner. You can consider strategies to use in managing your emerging responsibilities as well as choices you face as you assume the role of entry-level practitioner. You may become increasingly aware "that politics, ethics, paperwork, and a difficult pace, are part of practice" (Tyrssenaar & Perkins, 2001, p. 24). Using supervision to acknowledge these issues can help you learn to deal with them as you transition into your role as entry-level practitioner.

Delegating

In this final stage, your supervisor begins to delegate increased responsibility to you as you demonstrate heightened skill and comfort while meeting the role demands of an entry-level practitioner. The focus of supervision shifts from supporting your problem solving and decision making to monitoring and refining your work. You are more active in decision making and are essentially viewed by others as responsible for the OT service provision commensurate to your role. This phase of supervision often coincides with the final few weeks of a level II fieldwork experience, culminating in a final evaluation of your performance. This is ordinarily done using the Fieldwork Evaluation Form (AOTA, 1983, 1987). Feedback on the form is provided via a numerical rating of skill competencies outlined on the form accompanied by a narrative summary. These forms are under revision by the AOTA. Updated versions are expected to provide an easier mechanism for feedback, especially for fieldwork that occurs in emerging practice arenas.

You may again be asked by your supervisor to conduct a self-evaluation of your skills at the end of the experience. As mentioned earlier, for level II fieldwork, this is commonly done using the AOTA fieldwork evaluation forms or other reflective methods (i.e., written summary, questionnaire, checklist). It is important to prepare for the final evaluation session and the termination of the supervisory relationship. Prior to your evaluation meetings, you should complete a self-assessment to compare and contrast your impressions with your supervisor. You should be prepared as well to provide feedback to your supervisor about your experience. This is often done using the AOTA Student Evaluation of Fieldwork Form (Commission on Education, 2000). There is a specific section on the form for you to complete, with both a numerical rating scale and a section for narrative comments, regarding your supervisor/supervision.

As stated earlier, these four phases of supervision (directing, coaching, supporting, and delegating) are cyclical in nature. As the process evolves, through your growth and subsequently changing needs, your supervisor will most likely modify his or her approach and role. Should you encounter a new situation or new learning in which you feel challenged and in need of more support, coaching, or direction, your supervisor may temporarily revert to the style of supervision that coincides with your needs. The supervisory relationship should adjust accordingly as your skill acquisition and comfort level improve.

POSITIVE INFLUENCES ON THE SUPERVISORY PROCESS

Throughout the entire cycle of the supervisory relationship, three key elements of communication that support the process are the ability to listen, the ability to give and receive feedback, and conflict resolution skills.

Listening effectively involves viewing listening as a way to gather and use new information. When listening to someone, try to be aware of your own biases or immediate reactions that may be judgmental. Concentrate on what is being said, focusing your attention toward the content rather than the speaker's delivery. When you think the speaker is finished, restate the message in the form of a question, such as, "What I'm hearing you say is...," to make sure you comprehend the meaning. If you feel yourself reacting emotionally to what is being said, try to remain calm and look at the information as an opportunity to learn about, change, or rectify a situation.

Similarly, when receiving feedback, remember the purpose of feedback. Feedback is an avenue for receiving information about your actions and their effect on others. Feedback is a tool to let you know how you are performing and to suggest areas for improvement. Giving and receiving feedback in a constructive manner are skills that develop over time and can be refined with diligence and practice. Feedback is a mutual process involving both supervisor and supervisee.

When receiving feedback, it is important to stay open to hearing it. Try not to become defensive or interrupt. You and your supervisor are exchanging information. It may help to ask for specific examples, elaboration, or reminders about a given situation. You are seeking to understand your supervisor's point of view and to gather suggestions about a course of action, not debate or negate his or her statement. You should acknowledge positive feedback and choose an agreed-upon goal and timeline to make improvements in the areas discussed.

When giving feedback, timing is essential. Choose the right places and times to address concerns. Avoid letting issues build, or they may escalate to a conflict. You should focus your feedback on areas the individual can change. Feedback should address behaviors or activities, rather than personality traits. When giving feedback, you may want to follow a set framework to organize your approach. This involves using a statement with the components of "When you ___ I feel ___ because...," and following up your statement with questions such as, "What do you think?", "Do you agree?", or How do you feel about...?" to open up an opportunity for exchange. Feedback should be offered with examples, instead of generalizations, and in a way that demonstrates a desire to be helpful. Offering specific suggestions as to how the situation could be altered or improved is also necessary.

Barriers to giving and receiving feedback are often based in fear, uncertainty, or perceptions about your own competence. Fear may stem from being afraid of failure, not wanting to make the recipient of the feedback uncomfortable, or apprehension about being criticized. Questioning the approach to take in addressing the need for feedback, whether asking for, giving, or receiving feedback, can also be a stumbling block. Being overly confident or insecure about your skills is another potential obstacle to the feedback process.

Effective use of the feedback process in your supervisory relationship often helps to manage and resolve potential areas of conflict. Should conflicts escalate or remain unresolved, this can indicate an unwillingness to deal with conflicts directly. Individuals view situations from their own backgrounds, which can serve as a lens or filter for how they experience and interpret what is occurring. Life experience, ethics, values, and culture all play a role in the creation of this filter or lens. Realizing and appreciating that differences in opinions can exist and that at times there is no right or wrong answer is an important step in your professional development. If conflicting points of view are effectively resolved, innovative and creative solutions can be the result.

The following questions can aid you in taking steps to resolve conflict. They can serve as a template that can be used to help you evaluate the situation and guide you in the resolution process. When taking action to positively manage conflict, start by asking yourself the following questions:

➡ What are my past experiences with attempting to resolve conflict?

➡ Is the issue based on my relationship with this person?

➡ What are my current feelings about this person?

➡ How am I feeling about myself?

➡ How is my mood today? Am I anxious? Overwhelmed? Irritable? Disillusioned? Disempowered?

➡ How am I feeling physically? Tired? Tense?

➡ Could any of these variables be affecting my judgment?

➡ What do I see as the real issue that needs to be addressed?

➡ What are some possible solutions I could propose?

➡ Am I ready to take action and address this?

If you do not feel equipped to work toward a resolution, seek input from another professional within the organization or a resource person from your academic program who can serve as an impartial party and help you to view the situation from another perspective. Refrain from behaviors that are unprofessional, such as whining, gossiping, embellishing the issue, or bringing up extraneous complaints you may have been harboring. If you perceive that there are problems or issues to address, unless those involved are aware of them, they may not see any need for change or modifications, and the problem, along with your feelings about it, may continue to escalate. Working through conflict can be an opportunity for personal and professional growth. Staying neutral and non-judgmental can facilitate an open exchange about each party's needs and point of view. Focusing on the cause of the conflict and searching for solutions that are agreeable to all involved can strengthen the working alliance.

CONCLUSION

In closing, we would like to reiterate the importance of the supervisory process. The supervisory relationship is built upon a strong foundation. There are sequential steps to the formation of this mutual relationship, the outcome of which benefits all parties involved: you, your supervisor, and your clients. We hope that this information about the supervisory process, tasks, and roles; our exercises; as well as our personal narrative have been meaningful and are useful as you begin your professional journey. We trust that with your new knowledge and understanding, you will value the power of the supervisory relationship and process. Supervision can be an extraordi-

nary tool to keep you invested in your learning. The many personal and professional insights you may experience in supervision can energize and motivate you in your pursuit of your professional goals.

Supervision can help you to learn how to set realistic expectations of yourself and others as you face the many transitions and growth experiences that await you. It may be helpful to revisit this chapter and use the exercises repeatedly as you progress along the continuum of your professional development to your new role and identity as an entry-level practitioner in OT. We encourage you to apply the information learned about yourself in regard to communication styles, giving and receiving feedback, resolving conflict, and coping throughout your career. Exciting opportunities are ahead for you, and your potential can be maximized through a strong and effective supervisory relationship. Taking an active role in the relationship will be instrumental to your success.

REFERENCES

Accreditation Council for Occupational Therapy Education. (1998a). *Standards for an accredited educational program for the occupational therapist.* Bethesda, MD: The American Occupational Therapy Association, Inc.

Accreditation Council for Occupational Therapy Education. (1998b). *Standards for an accredited educational program for the occupational therapy assistant.* Bethesda, MD: The American Occupational Therapy Association, Inc.

American Occupational Therapy Association. (1983). *Fieldwork evaluation form for occupational therapy assistant students.* Bethesda, MD: Author.

American Occupational Therapy Association. (1987). *Fieldwork evaluation for the occupational therapist.* Bethesda, MD: Author.

Barnes, M. A., & Evenson, M. E. (1997). Fieldwork challenges. In K. Sladyk (Ed.), *The student primer: A guide to college success* (pp. 271-288). Thorofare, NJ: SLACK Incorporated.

Barnes, M. A., & Evenson, M. E. (2000). Structuring learning experiences. In S. C. Merrill & P. A. Crist (Eds.), *Meeting the fieldwork challenge: A self-paced clinical course, Lesson 6.* Bethesda, MD: The American Occupational Therapy Association, Inc.

Butler, H. F. (1972). Education for the professions: Student role stress. *Am J Occup Ther, 26,* 399-405.

Commission on Education. (2000). *Student evaluation of fieldwork experience.* Bethesda, MD: American Occupational Therapy Association.

Crist, P. (1996). Don't be a therapist to your student. *OT Practice, 1,* 15-17.

Crist, P., & McCarron, K. (2000). Supervision and mentoring. In S. C. Merrill & P. A. Crist (Eds.), *Meeting the fieldwork challenge: A self-paced clinical course, Lesson 5.* Bethesda, MD: The American Occupational Therapy Association, Inc.

Curtis, K. A. (1985). *Coaching for student success: Skills for the clinical instructor.* Los Angeles, CA: Health Directions, Educational Services for the Health Professions.

Ebb, W., McCoy, C., & Pugh, S. (1993). *Identifying the developmental needs of the fieldwork student.* Paper presented at The American Occupational Therapy Association, Inc. National Conference, Seattle, WA.

Herzberg, G. L. (1994). The successful fieldwork student: Supervisor perceptions. *Am J Occup Ther, 48,* 817-823.

Martin, H. H., & Martin, C. J. (1989). *Martin Operating Styles Inventory.* El Cajon, CA: Organization Improvement Systems.

Mitchell, M. M., & Kampfe, C. M. (1990). Coping strategies used by occupational therapy students during fieldwork: An exploratory study. *Am J Occup Ther, 44,* 543-550.

Sullivan, L. (1997). *Student fieldwork notebook.* Westboro, MA: UMASS Adolescent Program.

Tinson, A. (1999). Fieldwork task force compiles list of important characteristics of successful fieldwork students. *Student Voices, 10,* 1-2.

Tyrssenaar, J., & Perkins, J. (2001). From student to therapist: Exploring the first year of practice. *Am J Occup Ther, 55,* 19-27.

The authors would like to thank their reviewers, especially Mary Evenson, MPH, OTR, Dan Sullivan, and Lynne Sullivan, OTR/L.

Chapter 11

FIXING FIELDWORK PROBLEMS

Donna Whitehouse, MHA, OTR

Fieldwork is just about every student's favorite part of occupational therapy school. It is a time to apply things learned in the classroom, a time to interact with practicing therapists, and a time to work with "real" clients. Students look forward to this hands-on learning time with great anticipation. After all, this is what you are training for.

The last thing anybody wants to think about during this time is a fieldwork problem. But, unfortunately, problems can occur. The problem could be a personality issue between the student and the fieldwork educator; it could be that the student, for whatever reason, is not prepared for a particular type of experience; or a fieldwork educator is not adequately prepared for a student.

By the end of this chapter, you will do the following:

➡ Identify and list personal strengths and growth areas for clinical skills and professional behaviors.

➡ Review and understand how to deal with common fieldwork problems.

➡ Understand the characteristics of an effective student versus a challenging student.

➡ Understand the purpose of and how to use the "Tools for Fieldwork Success" in the fieldwork setting.

PREPARING FOR FIELDWORK

Before we discuss how to fix fieldwork problems, let us talk about how to proactively prepare for fieldwork. Reflection should begin in level I fieldwork as you plan level II fieldwork. Of course, you know that academic materials related to the practice area of your level II fieldwork experience should be reviewed. You may not be aware that you should also prepare for the "other half" of your professional life— the professional behaviors that can really make or break your fieldwork. By having a clear understanding of your strengths and growth areas in both clinical skills and professional behaviors, a student and fieldwork educator can work to design a fieldwork experience that can challenge the student and facilitate the growth of skills in both areas.

One of the first things a student should do for him- or herself in preparing for a fieldwork experience is to perform an honest self-appraisal of clinical skills and professional behaviors. This means sitting down and reflecting on your skills and identifying strengths and growth areas (see *Strengths and Growth Areas Worksheet* on p. 119). Ask a friend, fieldwork educators from level I fieldwork experiences, etc., to help you in this process. Once you have identified your fieldwork strengths and growth areas (here comes the intimidating part for some people), share them with your fieldwork educator. He or she will appreciate knowing the areas of knowledge in which you feel strong. He or she will also appreciate knowing where you would like to see some growth. He or she is not going to think any less of you because you have "growth areas." In fact, he or she is going to expect them. It will be much better for you as your fieldwork experience progresses if you have taken the time to develop this list and share this list with your fieldwork educator.

Case One

Laura was getting ready for her first level II. She had finished her academic coursework, and, although excited about her level IIs, she was also very anxious. During her 2 years of academic work, Laura had been through some pretty emotional times. Her father had died the week before school started, and now she was engaged to be married just after her fieldwork experience finished. She was pretty emotionally drained. During school, she knew that she was not her "old self" but thought things would be fine on fieldwork. She had been very quiet, did not participate much in class, and rarely smiled or laughed. She had a few friends, but mostly kept to herself. She had gotten feedback from her peers when doing academic group work that they would like to see her participate more in the discussions, planning, and presentation of assignments. Her instructors had also tried to point out that her affect and how much she participated really impacted her grade. Laura thought all would be fine once she got out on fieldwork.

Before she started fieldwork, Laura had talked with both her academic advisor and her academic fieldwork coordinator (AFWC). They asked how she was doing and what was she doing to prepare for fieldwork. Laura replied that she felt she was ready for level II, but hadn't done a whole lot to prepare beyond studying for classes. Laura and her AFWC discussed what they thought were Laura's strengths and growth areas. After identifying both, they discussed possible action plans for the growth areas. The AFWC suggested that Laura discuss with her fieldwork educator how she liked to give and get feedback. She also suggested that Laura tell her fieldwork educators that, although sometimes she might look disinterested, she really was interested in what she was learning. Laura needed to get into the habit of asking questions; she should let her fieldwork educator know that that was a goal of hers. Laura and her AFWC decided that she would ask her fieldwork educator to help her work on her goals of increasing initiation and participation in working with the clients. It was suggested that Laura talk to the fieldwork educator the first week about these issues so that there would be no "surprises." Laura stated that she thought these were good ideas and would talk to her fieldwork educator about working these goals into fieldwork.

Before she began fieldwork, Laura thought long and hard about what she should do. Even though she had agreed with her AFWC that she had some important goals to work on, she was really scared about sharing her "problems" with someone who would be grading her performance. She decided that she would not share her goals with the fieldwork educator as suggested. She decided that she would "wait and see." If she needed to bring these issues up later, she would, but she did not want the fieldwork educator to think that she had problems from the very first day.

On her third day of fieldwork, the fieldwork educator approached Laura. "Was she okay?" She did not seem interested in the work, she did not ask any questions, and she did not ask to try her hand at a treatment session. Laura said she was fine. By the end of the week, the fieldwork educator was calling Laura's AFWC to ask for help because Laura seemed only to give a half-hearted effort to her work. By the end of the second week, there was discussion about possibly needing to end the fieldwork experience. When the AFWC spoke with Laura about her field-

STRENGTHS AND GROWTH AREAS WORKSHEET

Strengths (Examples)	*Growth Areas (Examples)*
Good time management skills	Need to work on being more assertive in asking questions when I'm unsure of what I'm being asked to do
Organized	I get embarrassed when I get constructive feedback in front of others
I get along well with other students and staff members	Sometimes I am too hard on myself when I make a mistake
I feel very strong in my knowledge of anatomical structures	I have difficulty figuring out what types of treatment activities would be good for different types of clients
I have a good understanding of psychiatric diagnoses and common medications	I am not sure how to handle a difficult or unruly client
I work well with children	My transfer skills are pretty weak
Strengths	*Growth Areas*
_____	_____
_____	_____
_____	_____
_____	_____
_____	_____

work experience, she asked if Laura had shared the discussed goals with her fieldwork educator. Laura said, no, she did not want anyone to think that there was a problem.

WHAT HAPPENS IF...

As students prepare for fieldwork, they often have a list of "what if" questions. The following list has been prepared as a quick reference for frequently asked questions. Note: School policy and procedure should be followed in every situation. The following are suggestions only and do not override school or fieldwork site protocol.

What happens if...

Everything Is Fine

➡ Call your AFWC at the school and tell him or her. Most schools have a policy or procedure about checking in around midterm; they might do a site visit as well. All AFWCs love to hear that things are going well, that you are enjoying the experience, and that you are learning a lot.

I See Unethical Things Being Practiced

➡ Do not automatically assume that you have interpreted the observed situation accurately. Call a trusted mentor to discuss. This could be your AFWC, an advisor at school, etc. Students should seek clarification on the issue from the fieldwork educator before drawing conclusions.

Yes, this can be intimidating. If you determine that you need to take action, the questioning approach can be along the lines of "I observed _____ yesterday, and I am confused. I do not understand why that happened. Could you please clarify for me?" If the answer to this query clears up your question, then there is no need to proceed further. If you are still not satisfied with the answer, there are several steps to take.

➡ Ask again, just to make sure that you are certain about what you have seen.

➡ Tell your fieldwork educator that you are feeling uncomfortable with the approach being used and would like to discuss the policy with the next up in the chain of command.

➡ Discuss the situation with your AFWC.

➡ If all involved determine that the action is questionable or unethical, then your AFWC will need to work with the site and you to determine the next course of action. This could include but is not limited to changing the fieldwork educator, switching to another program at the fieldwork site, or being removed from the fieldwork site.

Dealing with questionable ethics is very difficult for anyone—student or practicing therapists. The above-described approach is direct and can be intimidating to carry through. Students must remember that they are learning how to be professionals, and one of the most important characteristics of any effective professional is the ability to address a situation openly and honestly.

Case Two

Zoë was in her first week of her first level II. She was working at a small hospital and was excited about finally getting full-time hands-on learning. On her second day, Zoë was learning about documentation. She was reading over her fieldwork educator's notes from the previous day and noted that some treatment details were recorded differently from what she had remembered seeing. The amount of time recorded for the patient's session was about twice as long as the patient had actually been in treatment. The patient's level of performance was also listed as significantly higher than what Zoë had observed. Confused, Zoë decided to watch treatments that day and review documentation again for the day's treatment. Maybe she was missing something.

Unfortunately, when Zoë reviewed the day's documentation, she again found that her observations did not match up with the written note of her fieldwork educator. Zoë contacted her AFWC. The AFWC was

concerned, but also knew that sometimes students' understanding of a treatment or procedure differed from the fieldwork educator's perspective due to policies of the site, different practice techniques, etc. The AFWC recommended that Zoë address her concerns with her fieldwork educator. Zoë was very nervous; she did not want to accuse her fieldwork educator of any wrong doing, but her concerns over what she was seeing really wouldn't allow her to keep silent. Zoë asked, "I was reviewing documentation yesterday and noticed that the information written did not exactly match what we did in treatment, and I'm not sure why. Could you help me understand?" To Zoë's great surprise, her fieldwork educator acknowledged that the documentation was different than the treatment session. The fieldwork educator stated that the patient was not showing much improvement. For the hospital to get paid, she needed to show improvement, so she documented that the patient was doing better than she really was. Zoë was shocked to say the least. She contacted her AFWC, who was also alarmed. The AFWC made a visit to the site, asked the fieldwork educator the same questions about documentation, and received the same answer. Due to the fact that the fieldwork educator was documenting services illegally and unethically, Zoë was removed from the fieldwork site and finished her fieldwork at a different location.

I Get Hurt or Become Sick

➡ Should you get an injury or become ill while at work, first, follow the program/facility guidelines and obtain the appropriate medical services. If necessary and appropriate, contact family/friends, etc.

➡ If you are hurt or become ill outside of fieldwork hours, first seek appropriate medical attention. After you have been cared for and the physician has instructed you on activity restrictions (if any), contact both your fieldwork educator and your AFWC. The fieldwork educator and AFWC will determine the impact of this illness or injury on the fieldwork experience.

➡ If you are using your school's insurance plan as your medical coverage, you will need to contact your Student Health Office and let them know of the situation. Check with your school on their policies for off-campus medical emergencies.

➡ Contact your school and let them know what happened, how you are, and the impact this might have on your fieldwork experience.

➡ Should your fieldwork experience need to be delayed for any reason due to injury or illness, you, your fieldwork educator, and the AFWC will need to discuss possible options to make up time. Any changes in the fieldwork experience should involve a discussion with all parties; students should not make decisions about their fieldwork timeline independent of the school.

I Have a Family Emergency

➡ If you are contacted about an emergency at work, talk with your fieldwork educator about your needs and concerns. Together, you will need to determine, for the immediate future, what the plan of action will be.

➡ If you are contacted about an emergency after work hours and cannot make it to work the next day, contact your fieldwork educator either at home or first thing in the morning. If possible, it is best to talk directly with the fieldwork educator and not leave a message. If you need to leave a message, call back later to make sure that the message was received.

➡ At some point, contact your school and apprise them of the situation. If you are unable to call the school, ask your fieldwork educator to contact them for you. Once the situation has stabilized, contact your AFWC to discuss how long you need to be away from fieldwork and other pertinent information. The school and the fieldwork site will make decisions on what will happen with the fieldwork experience after discussion with the student.

There Is a Natural Disaster or Emergency Situation at My Fieldwork Site

➡ Seek shelter, following the policies and procedures of the fieldwork site.

➡ Seek medical attention as needed. Follow same steps as described above if you are injured.

➡ If/when possible, get word to family and school to let them know what has happened and your condition.

Case Three

George and Julia were at their level I fieldwork in Seattle. Things were going fine, and they were learning a lot. All of the sudden, George looked up, and the lights were swinging back and forth. Julia looked down, and the floor seemed to be moving. Back home, their parents were watching television, and a news flash came on ("Earthquake in Seattle"—a picture of George and Julia's fieldwork site came on the news). At the same time, a news flash came on the radio of the AFWC of their school. The only pictures and information getting back to the school were that serious damage had been done, but they were unsure of the amount.

George and Julia first followed the procedures of the fieldwork site as directed by their fieldwork educators. Once all was clear, they tried to call home. Realizing that phone access was limited, they contacted their school, told the AFWC that they were fine, and asked that she contact their families. Their families were very relieved to hear that they were both okay.

There Is a Labor Strike

➡ Contact your AFWC and follow procedures as directed.

➡ If your school does not have procedures for a labor strike the following is recommended: If your fieldwork educator is going in to work, make plans to go into work as well. But, if, at any point in time, you feel that you are not physically safe, turn back and do not attempt to cross the picket lines. If it appears that the strike will be lasting an indefinite period of time, you, your fieldwork instructor, and your AFWC will talk about the future of your fieldwork at this site and discuss alternatives.

I Do Not Like My Fieldwork Educator

In a working relationship, personal feelings about a coworker or fieldwork educator need to be kept in check. You may have different views about politics, religion, life choices, etc., but these are personal opinions that should not enter into a working relationship. Is it easy to ignore? No. But, especially for a student, you are not there to debate the pros and cons of the latest Supreme Court decision. You are at the fieldwork site to learn. The first thing that you need to figure out is if you can learn from your fieldwork educator. If the answer is yes, then you need to overcome your own personal feelings about subject matter that does not relate to the fieldwork experience and forge ahead with the learning opportunity you have been given.

As with most difficult situations, the best approach (and often the most intimidating) is the direct approach. Talk with your fieldwork educator about your concerns of student/fieldwork educator compatibility. Give that fieldwork educator the opportunity to make some changes. Consider your role in the relationship. Be prepared to get constructive feedback on your working style, and be prepared to make changes in your approach to the fieldwork experience.

Keep in mind that this fieldwork experience is not forever. If you can make it work, then do that. If you feel like you and your fieldwork educator really cannot get along, then explore other options. If another fieldwork educator is available, consider requesting a change. Remember, just as you want to know what you are doing right or wrong, your fieldwork educator needs to get that feedback as well. Do not show up one day requesting a change in fieldwork educators. Make sure that you have gone through the proper channels and that your fieldwork educator is aware of your frustrations and agrees that this is the best idea in order for you to have a successful experience.

There Are Other Students at This Site, and I Do Not Get Along With One/Some/All of Them

This is a working relationship. You should handle the situation just like you would if you were an employee. Try to find common areas or interests for you and the other student to explore. If you find there is nothing in common or your work styles do not mesh and you are having difficulty getting your job done, discuss it with your fieldwork educator. Again, you do not have to personally like someone to work effectively with him or her.

I Do Not Think the Fieldwork Educator Is Competent In His or Her Practice Area

This is not an easy situation. The first thing you need to figure out is whether you can learn in that environment. If you can learn and contribute to the setting, then see if you can make it work for the remainder of your experience. If you do not think you can learn in the practice environment, there are some options.

➡ First, your fieldwork educator needs to know that you have concerns. Do not surprise him or her with the fact that you are not happy. You do not have to say, "I think you are incompetent," but

you do need to address the issue. You can ask questions such as, "I'm not sure I understand the rationale behind that approach. Could you explain?" or "I have read about ____, which is different from what you are doing. Can you help me understand the differences?" You may find that you have underestimated the fieldwork educator or that you do not have a full grasp of the situation.

➡ If, after discussion with your fieldwork educator and AFWC, you still feel that you cannot learn in the current environment, you can request a change in fieldwork educators if one is available or request a withdrawal altogether from the experience. Withdrawal from an experience has many ramifications and is not something that a student on fieldwork can decide without discussion with the fieldwork educator and AFWC.

My Fieldwork Educator Quits While I Am There

Do not panic! Most places will develop a back-up plan for situations like this. Either there is another therapist with whom you can work or there is another location within their system to which you can transfer. Your fieldwork educator should contact the AFWC at your school to inform him or her of the situation and to review options for the continuation of your fieldwork experience.

My Fieldwork Site Does Not Practice OT the Way I Was Taught

All practitioners are called on to follow the Standards Practice as outlined in *The Guide to Occupational Therapy Practice* (Moyers, 1997). Within this framework, there is a lot of leeway in how services are actually delivered. If the fieldwork site does not practice OT the way you were taught, there are typically two reasons why. First, OT schools work very hard to provide you with training in the latest advances in rehabilitation. These advances are perfected in the practice setting. If your school did not teach you a particular approach or technique, it may be that the approach is new or in the process of being developed—a great opportunity for you take advantage of while on fieldwork. Second, the philosophy toward client care may be very different at your fieldwork site when compared to your school. Your school may teach you to be very client centered and to use a holistic approach when developing interventions. On the flip side, your fieldwork site may practice through one frame of reference with all clients. For example, the therapists at your fieldwork site may have a biomechanical approach to interventions, such as exercising or cone placement. If you find yourself in this dilemma, discuss the differences in what you have been taught and what you are seeing in practice with both your fieldwork educator and your AFWC. The information you get from your AFWC and fieldwork educator should help you balance out the discrepancies you are seeing in practice.

A word of caution: if you are told, "well, this is how its done in the real world," be careful. A good fieldwork site combines many different educational and treatment approaches. There is no one way to do the right thing. A good therapist will stay open to new ideas and treatment approaches throughout his or her career.

By the same token, you have to be ready to bend and mold yourself to the situation as appropriate. You may be very clear on how an activity or intervention should be performed and still be told that you need to modify your approach. If you find that you have difficulty modifying, consider that it may not be the fieldwork site that has a problem; it may be you.

If you find yourself in a situation in which you cannot seem to resolve the differences in what you were taught and what is in practice on fieldwork, discuss your issues with your AFWC and your fieldwork educator. Determine what options are available for the remainder of your experience.

I Am On a "Nontraditional" Fieldwork Site, and the OT Is Not With Me Very Often

The Accreditation Committee on Occupational Therapy Education (American Occupational Therapy Association [AOTA], 1998a, 1998b) states that, for level I fieldwork, educators can be selected from any number of professionals. These can include, but are not limited to, occupational therapy practitioners, legislators, physicians, teachers, social workers, nurses, physical therapists, and recreational or activity therapists (AOTA, 1998a, 1998b). For level II experiences when an OT practitioner is not on site, a plan for the provision of occupational therapy services must be documented and provided to the student, school, and fieldwork site. When on-site supervision is provided, it must be in accordance with the plan and meet state credentialing guidelines. In this type of setting, both the OT and OTA student must receive a minimum of 6 hours of occupational therapy supervision per week. This includes direct observation of client interaction. During all working hours, the occupational therapy fieldwork educator must be readily available for communication and/or consultation if needed (AOTA, 1998a, 1998b).

If you are working in a setting with no OT or little OT contact, make sure that you know to whom to go when you have OT questions. If you are on a level I experience and have a question about what an OT might do with a particular client, ask your level I fieldwork educator to get his or her perspective, or call your school to discuss with a faculty member. If you are on level II, the supervision plan should outline whom to contact when you have a question about service delivery and occupational therapy in general.

I Am the Primary Caregiver for My Children, Parents, Grandparents, Etc.

You should take steps to make sure that they are taken care of while you're on fieldwork, but sometimes they will get sick and need you at home. Situations like this warrant open and honest discussion with your fieldwork educator. Your fieldwork educator needs to know that you have outside obligations that may impact your attendance at fieldwork. Prior to talking with your fieldwork educator, prepare a list of options to cover your caregiver obligations should you not be able to leave work and prepare a list of options to get your work covered if you need to leave work. Such options can include, but are not limited to, working on Saturdays, working extended evening hours, and working beyond the planned 12 weeks. Share this information with your fieldwork educator. This type of planning shows him or her that you are committed to the fieldwork experience and want to make sure that you participate as a full member of the team.

Some fieldwork sites and/or schools allow you to miss a certain number of days without making time up. Others state that you are required to attend fieldwork 100% of the time, no absences allowed. Check the policy with your school prior to leaving for fieldwork. AOTA policy on absences is as follows: "Time off during fieldwork is decided by the fieldwork site and the academic program. You should direct any questions about taking time off to your academic fieldwork coordinator and/or fieldwork educator" (AOTA, 2000).

I Do Not Agree With the Marks That I've Been Given on My Evaluation

Evaluating a student on fieldwork is not easy. There is much time, thought, and effort that goes into completing an evaluation. The fieldwork educator is the expert while on your fieldwork experience. His or her judgment needs to be respected. There is a reason why he or she has that opinion of you and your work. Figure out why that is, and move on from there.

In the event of a personality clash between student and fieldwork educator and either the student or fieldwork educator feels that the poor personal relationship might interfere with the evaluation of performance, the AFWC should be contacted as soon as possible. A discussion should occur with all parties and an action plan developed to address the personality issues.

I'm Failing At Midterm

The first 4 to 6 weeks of your fieldwork experience are an orientation and exposure time to get you up to speed to carry your own caseload. If you are having difficulty at the halfway mark, you really need to hit the books hard and do whatever it takes to pull yourself out of danger. If you are in trouble at midterm, your fieldwork educator should contact your AFWC and discuss the current situation. You should contact your AFWC on your own after discussing the issues with the fieldwork educator. If your fieldwork location is not within travel distance for an on-site meeting, you, your fieldwork educator, and your AFWC might have a phone conference call to discuss options. Your school will have its own policies and procedures on how to handle failing marks at midterm. Refer to that information for specifics.

I Am Asked To Leave/Withdraw From An Experience

Each school has its own policies on how fieldwork withdrawal and termination are handled. Refer to Chapter 12 for information on dealing with withdrawal and termination. Keep in mind that this is a learning experience. Remember to maintain professional behaviors so that leaving is a positive experience for all involved.

I Failed One Fieldwork Experience

Each school has its own policies on how fieldwork withdrawal and termination are handled. Refer to Chapter 12 for information on dealing with with-

drawal and termination. Contact your AFWC for further guidance, and set up an appointment back at school to review the experience. Use the time before this meeting to reflect on the experience and to develop an action plan to address issues identified by your fieldwork educator. Be proactive.

I Failed Two Fieldwork Experiences

Each school has its own policies on how fieldwork withdrawal and termination are handled. Refer to Chapter 12 for information on dealing with withdrawal and termination. Remember that a second failure may mean graduating with a degree other than occupational therapy.

Effective vs. Challenging Student

Students bring many things with them to their fieldwork experience: books, notes, lab coats, etc. Perhaps two of the most important things students bring to the placement are their personality and work ethic. Research has shown that students with a positive attitude toward their work are evaluated as having a higher degree of clinical skills than students with an expressed negative attitude (Tickle-Degnen & Puccinelli, 1999). How you approach your work significantly impacts how you and the outcome of your efforts are perceived.

Students are not expected to be "perfect." They are expected to try hard, be academically prepared, and be ready to learn. The comparison chart in *Effective Student vs. Challenging Student Comparison* delineates the differences between an effective student and a challenging student. At any point in time, a student could exhibit characteristics on either list. Students should strive to have more traits on the "effective" list, especially as the fieldwork progresses. If you note that you are having problems, especially problems similar to the "challenging" student, talk with your fieldwork educator.

Tools for Fieldwork Success

A successful fieldwork experience requires planning, effort, time, and attention to detail. The following worksheets are recommended as tools to help you facilitate a great fieldwork. They can be used when things are going well, and they can be used when things are not so great. Their purpose is to open lines of communication and outline expectations of performance.

EFFECTIVE STUDENT VS. CHALLENGING STUDENT COMPARISON

Effective Student	*Challenging Student*
Asks questions, speaks to others	Withdrawn
Energetic, cheerful	Depressed attitude
Honest, forthright	Manipulative
Listens carefully to feedback and participates in the problem-solving process	Has an excuse for most problems
Does not discuss the strengths and growth areas of others beyond appropriate conversations	Projects own problems onto others
Continuously monitors own performance and seeks feedback from a variety of sources	Poor insight
Develops personal system for organization of tasks and assignments	Poor organizational skills
Asks questions of others when needing assistance, independently monitors caseload, assignments, etc.	Requires a lot of outside pressure to keep up with minimum standards
Seeks feedback from fieldwork educator, shows initiative in trying new tasks, aware of growth areas but not afraid to try new things	Heavy reliance on fieldwork educator
Assignments and job tasks are completed in a timely manner	Work is consistently late, incomplete, and/or not up to set standards
Honest	Dishonest
Is open to hearing constructive feedback and seeks clarification on issues not fully understood	Defensive when given constructive feedback
Calm, cool, and collected	Hostile
Appreciates the time, energy, and efforts put forth by fieldwork site and fieldwork educator	Arrogant
Flexible	Critical of department, staff, procedures
Seeks clarification if unsure about performing new tasks, does not hesitate to perform routine tasks	Does not initiate tasks independently
Manages routine tasks effectively, initiates discussion with fieldwork educator if having difficulty completing assignments	Often overwhelmed
Gives 110% effort	Attempts to "get by" but falls short
Academically prepared, spends own time after work as needed preparing for fieldwork	Poorly prepared and cannot seem to "catch up" on the job *(continued)*

Effective Student vs. Challenging Student Comparison (Continued)

Effective Student	Challenging Student
On time for work, completes paperwork and assignments on time, maintains client schedule	Unreliable
Learns from mistakes, asks questions, initiates discussion if unsure of how to complete task	Makes same mistakes repeatedly, regardless of how many times discussed
Is aware of strengths and growth areas. Modifies performance after feedback. Critiques own performance, finding both strengths and growth areas with minimal prompting	Extremely self-critical
Supports school and/or uses professional language when critiquing program	Criticizes school
Keeps a personal issue away from work. If having personal difficulty that interrupts work, discreetly discusses problems with fieldwork educator	Emotional over-reactions: both work and nonwork-related
Completes assigned work in a timely manner. While at fieldwork site, concentrates on work-related activities	Appears "busy," but not with work-related tasks
Rested	Always tired
Is friendly to staff and patients	Does not get along with other students and staff
Requires close supervision at beginning of fieldwork. As fieldwork progresses, supervision can be pulled back due to the increasing level of independent performance	Requires constant supervision for entire fieldwork experience
Talks with fieldwork educator when unsure of self or skills, or when wants to explore a new/different area of intervention	Does not communicate learning needs
Follows schedule, attends meetings, mingles well with other staff	Cannot seem to "get into" the routine
Gets along well with patients, directs intervention so that client feels that "personal touch" has been given and goals are met	Spends more time socializing with patients than treating them
Is aware of safety hazards and precautions	Poor safety judgment
Delivers effective therapeutic interventions	Can verbalize ideas but not carry out effectively
Progresses patients, in a timely manner, toward their long-term goals	Difficulty working with patients toward their long-term goals
Takes responsibility for own learning needs	Does not take responsibility for self or learning experience

Adapted from Bird, C., & Aukas, R. (1998). *Meeting the fieldwork challenge: Strategies for a new century*. Professional Development Program sponsored by the Continuing Education Department, American Occupational Therapy Association.

STUDENT/FIELDWORK EDUCATOR WEEKLY REVIEW

Week # _____
Strengths:

Growth areas:

Goals for the upcoming week:

Meetings, assignments, etc.:

Student signature _____ Date _____

Supervisor signature _____ Date _____

Student/Fieldwork Educator Weekly Review

Students and fieldwork educators should have a planned time during the week to sit down privately and review the past week's performance. Using the worksheet (see *Student/Fieldwork Educator Weekly Review*), strengths and noticeable gains should be discussed, as well as an objective critique of performance and what needs to be improved. Students should prepare a self-critique separate from their fieldwork educator, and both should share at the weekly meeting.

Learning Contracts

A learning contract is a written document that is jointly developed by the student and the fieldwork educator (Gaiptman & Anthony, 1989). The document is based on the learning objectives of the school and fieldwork site, and the contract individualizes the students' fieldwork experience and outlines the responsibilities of both the student and fieldwork educator (Gaiptman & Anthony, 1989). The student and supervising therapist develop the learning contract together, using the worksheet (see *Learning Contract* on p. 128) with the goal of addressing the core skills of a therapist at the fieldwork site while tailoring experiences when possible to the students' learning style and interests (see *Sample Learning Contract* on p. 128). The learning contract can be used in conjunction with the *Strengths and Growth Areas Worksheet* (p. 119).

Professional Behaviors Competence Document

Fieldwork success or failure is not totally determined by clinical competence. Students must be active members of the team. They must communicate well with others, show initiative, and have good problem-solving abilities. These "professional behaviors," while critical to performance, can be difficult to measure. The *Professional Behaviors Competence Document* worksheet (p. 129) is designed to evaluate the professional behaviors of a student, requires specific examples of the behavior in question, and asks for remediation ideas (see *Remediation Ideas* on p. 130). It can be scored for performance on level I or level II (see *Washington University School of Medicine Program in Occupational Therapy Level I and Level II Fieldwork Evaluation Supplements* on pp. 131-132).

Strengths and Growth Areas Worksheet

A competent professional constantly reviews his or her performance, looking for areas that have improved or that could be improved. An appraisal such as this takes into account the individual's own personal judgment of performance and requests feedback from others. To effectively address the development of the identified growth areas, it is recommended that the student share his or her strengths and growth area worksheet (p. 119) with his or her field-

---

LEARNING CONTRACT

What do I need/want to know?
What resources will I use to find out what I need/want to know?
How will what I know be evaluated and by whom?
Completion date

SAMPLE LEARNING CONTRACT

➡ *What do I need/want to know?*
  To make one static and one dynamic splint for clients with no mistakes.
➡ *What resources will I use to find out what I need/want to know?*
  Review splinting with fieldwork educator; get materials to practice different types of splints; observe other therapists; review notes from school; practice making different types of splints and have others critique.
➡ *How will what I know be evaluated and by whom?*
  I will be evaluated by my supervising therapist and by my patient. Fieldwork educator must agree that the splint is appropriate for the patient, is technically correct, and must agree with my prescribed wearing plan. The patient must agree that the splint fits appropriately, is comfortable, and must be able to don/doff independently.
➡ *Completion Date*
  By midterm of fieldwork.

---

work educator and develop fieldwork goals to address both the strengths and the growth areas. Note: The Strengths and Growth Areas Worksheet can be used in conjunction with the *Learning Contract*.

SUMMARY

I find that when I talk about fieldwork issues with my students, the issues I discuss tend to be about fieldwork problems—about what goes wrong, "battlefield" stories, and how they were overcome, etc. I have learned from my students that I need to end our discussions with an uplifting note, reminding them that while we discuss the nitty gritty about what can go wrong, generally, everything really is going to be all right.

I have found that both academically strong and weak students can do well on fieldwork, and both can do poorly. I have found that any student can be an excellent therapist when he or she is motivated to succeed. I have found that if a student is resilient, no matter his or her background, grades, or anything else, that student can be successful in meeting the challenges that come his or her way.

REFERENCES

American Occupational Therapy Association. (1998a). *Standards for the accreditation of educational programs for the occupational therapist. The reference manual of the official documents of the American Occupational Therapy Association, Inc.* Bethesda, MD: Author.

American Occupational Therapy Association. (1998b). *Standards for the accreditation of educational programs for the occupational therapy assistant. The reference manual of the official documents of the American Occupational Therapy Association, Inc.* Bethesda, MD: Author.

American Occupational Therapy Association. (2000). *AOTA fieldwork information for students: Most frequently asked questions.* www.aota.org.

Gaiptman, B., & Anthony, A. (1989). Contracting in fieldwork education: The model of self-directed learning. *Can J Occup Ther, 56,* 10-14.

Moyers, P. (1997). *The guide to occupational therapy practice.* Bethesda, MD: American Occupational Therapy Association.

Tickle-Degnen, L., & Puccinelli, N. (1999). The nonverbal expression of negative emotions: Peer and fieldwork educator responses to occupational therapy students' emotional attributes. *The Occupational Therapy Journal of Research, 19,* 18-39.

PROFESSIONAL BEHAVIORS COMPETENCE DOCUMENT

Professional Behaviors: Does the Individual Exhibit...	Yes	Needs Improvement	No	N/A
Positive Attitude				
—Fosters positive communication	5	3	0	5
—Accepts change	5	3	0	5
—Manages stressors in positive and constructive ways	5	2	0	5
Flexibility				
—Can adapt and cope with change	5	3	0	5
—Modifies performance after feedback	5	2	0	5
Professional communication skills				
—Practices positive verbal and nonverbal interpersonal communication skills in work interactions	5	3	0	5
—Is concise in verbal and written communication	5	3	0	5
—Handles conflict constructively	5	3	0	5
—Uses assertive communication skills	5	3	0	5
—Written communication demonstrates correct grammar, spelling, punctuation, etc.	5	3	0	5
A willingness to "go the extra mile"				
—Seeks ways to improve	5	3	0	5
—Volunteers for additional responsibilities	5	3	0	5
—Takes on additional responsibilities	5	3	0	5
Respect of others				
—Follows the chain of command	5	3	0	5
—Is supportive of others	5	3	0	5
—Can listen to other viewpoints—whether agree or disagree	5	3	0	5
—Respects diversity	5	2	0	5
—Attentive to guests' needs	5	3	0	5
—Is sensitive to others' timeframes	5	3	0	5
—Meets deadlines; if unable to meet deadline, informs necessary parties and schedules new deadline	5	3	0	5
A "team player" attitude				
—Strives to achieve team goals	5	2	0	5
—Is proactive and anticipates needs of others	5	3	0	5
—Pools resources and works efficiently within a group	5	3	0	5
—Assists with resolution development after problem is identified	5	3	0	5
Personal responsibility				
—Is aware of strengths and weaknesses	5	3	0	5
—Punctual	5	3	0	5
—Demonstrates initiative	5	3	0	5
—Follows safety precautions	5	3	0	5
—Respects and maintains confidentiality	5	3	0	5
—Demonstrates an awareness of/follows the Code of Ethics	5	3	0	5

PROFESSIONAL BEHAVIORS COMPETENCE DOCUMENT (CONTINUED)

Professional Behaviors: Does the Individual Exhibit...	Yes	Needs Improvement	No	N/A
Appropriate dress and hygiene				
—Follows program guidelines	5	3	0	5

Yes: The individual exhibits these behaviors a minimum of 90% of the time.
Needs Improvement: Exhibits behaviors 50% to 89% of the time, but needs improvement.
No: The individual exhibits these behaviors less than 50% of the time.
All "Inconsistent" and "No" marks should be identified through examples.

Developed by Donna Whitehouse, MHA, OTR; Chris Ahr, OTR; Debbie Dinzebach, OTR; and Jan Duchek, PhD.

©1998 Whitehouse, Duchek, Ahr, and Dinzebach and reprinted with permission of Washington University School of Medicine Program in Occupational Therapy.

REMEDIATION IDEAS

Each "Needs Improvement" and "No" mark should be documented through examples. Recommendations for improvement are appreciated. Students will meet with the Coursemaster of the Professional Practice class for areas needing improvement. Action plans incorporating the suggestions of each fieldwork site will be developed at the school in an effort to address areas identified.

1. Item:
Example:
Recommendation:

2. Item:
Example:
Recommendation:

3. Item:
Example:
Recommendation:

4. Item:
Example:
Recommendation:

5. Item:
Example:
Recommendation:

Comments:

Student Signature _____ Date _____

Fieldwork Educator Signature _____ Date _____

WASHINGTON UNIVERSITY SCHOOL OF MEDICINE PROGRAM IN OCCUPATIONAL THERAPY LEVEL I FIELDWORK EVALUATION SUPPLEMENT

Student Name:

Date(s) of Experience:

Program:

Fieldwork Educator:

Total Evaluation Score: _____ (155 points total)

Minimum Scores:
First Level I Fieldwork:	108
Second Level I Fieldwork:	108
Third Level I Fieldwork:	116
Fourth Level I Fieldwork:	124

The purpose of a level I fieldwork experience is to provide an opportunity for exposure to occupational therapy intervention and programming or, in the cases where no OT services are currently being provided, exposure to potential growth areas for OT. We encourage as much "hands on" as possible and appropriate within each experience.

Our evaluation is designed to monitor and evaluate the progress the student makes toward a working health care professional. Opportunities for the student to carry out interventions will vary from site to site. The Washington University Program in Occupational Therapy feels that regardless of the amount of "hands on" opportunities the student has during the experience, the expectation for professional behaviors should be the same.

The Professional Behaviors Competence Document outlines eight major categories of professional behavior. Within each category, there are specific behaviors to be rated. A score of "YES" indicates that the behavior is exhibited 90% to 100% of the time. A score of "NEEDS IMPROVEMENT" indicates that the student demonstrates the identified behavior 50% to 89% of the time. If the student demonstrates an identified behavior less than 50% of the time, the score should be marked as "NO." We recognize that all behaviors may not be observed or demonstrated during a fieldwork experience. In that situation, a score of "N/A" would be marked. If a student receives an "N/A" score, he or she is not penalized, as it carries the same numerical weight as a "YES" score.

For each behavior rated "NEEDS IMPROVEMENT" or "NO," an example should be provided as well as a recommendation for improvement. The evaluation and recommendations should be reviewed with the student at the fieldwork site. These remarks again will be reviewed at the school and, when needed, will be followed by a discussion with the student.

Thank you for your participation in our program and your assistance in the educational process of our occupational therapy students.

WASHINGTON UNIVERSITY SCHOOL OF MEDICINE PROGRAM IN OCCUPATIONAL THERAPY LEVEL II FIELDWORK EVALUATION SUPPLEMENT

Student Name:

Date(s) of Experience:

Program:

Fieldwork Educator:

Total Evaluation Score: _____ (155 points total)

Minimum Scores: Midterm: 132
                             Final: 140

This evaluation supplement is designed to highlight the growth of professional behavior skills during the Level II fieldwork experience. It is suggested that this form be utilized at midterm and at final evaluations. Scores have been set to reflect expected performance of an entry-level therapist by the final evaluation.

The Professional Behaviors Competence Document outlines eight major categories of professional behavior. Within each category, there are specific behaviors to be rated. A score of "YES" indicates that the behavior is exhibited 90% to 100% of the time. A score of "NEEDS IMPROVEMENT" indicates that the student demonstrates the identified behavior 50% to 89% of the time. If the student demonstrates an identified behavior less than 50% of the time, the score should be marked as "NO." We recognize that all behaviors may not be observed or demonstrated during a fieldwork experience. In that situation, a score of "N/A" would be marked. If a student receives an "N/A" score, he or she is not penalized, as it carries the same numerical weight as a "YES" score.

For each behavior rated "NEEDS IMPROVEMENT" or "NO," an example should be provided as well as a recommendation for improvement. The evaluation and recommendations should be reviewed with the student at the fieldwork site. These remarks again will be reviewed at the school and, when needed, be followed by a discussion with the student.

Thank you for your participation in our program and for your assistance in the educational process of our occupational therapy students.

©1998 Whitehouse, Duchek, Ahr, Dinzenbach and reprinted with permission of Washington University School of Medicine Program in Occupational Therapy.

Chapter 12

DEALING WITH WITHDRAWAL OR TERMINATION

Linda Duncombe, EdD, OTR, FAOTA

No one likes to think about the possibility of withdrawing from or terminating an internship. One looks forward to an internship as being the highlight of one's academic career, a learning experience, and a confidence-builder. McCarron and Crist (2000) refer to fieldwork as a capstone experience. When, for whatever reason, the fieldwork experience cannot be completed, students may question what they learned from the experience and may begin to doubt their ability to become an occupational therapy practitioner (Kyler-Hutchison, 1994).

All of life is a process and a learning experience, not an end product. Successes and failures are part of that experience (Ilott, 1995). By the end of the chapter, you will realize the following:

➡ There are many reasons for a withdrawal or termination.

➡ There are aspects of the fieldwork experience from which you learned and you grew as a person and as a professional.

➡ There are no negative experiences, only learning experiences.

Withdrawals are frequently initiated by the student or the academic program. Terminations are usually requested by the facility. The main reasons for withdrawals are personal illness, serious illness, or death of a family member, or a feeling on the part of the student that the pace at the facility is too fast or that the supervisor's personality is so different from his or her own that he or she is unable to communicate. When a facility suggests termination of a student, the student is probably not passing the internship and has not met the requirements of the learning contract, and the supervisor feels the student needs time to build skills, work on judgment, or change his or her attitude before continuing. Sometimes, a supervisor feels that a different type of setting would be a better match for the student.

When either withdrawal or termination is recommended, the decision to remove the student from the fieldwork experience is well thought-out. Ilott (1995) refers to it as a "soul-searching" experience. In other words, the decision is not reached lightly or impulsively.

Withdrawal

If there are issues in your personal life that make it difficult for you to concentrate on your internship, or if for any reason you feel it might be necessary to withdraw, contact your academic fieldwork coordinator (AFWC) immediately. Sometimes, students are feeling overwhelmed, and the AFWC can help put concerns in perspective and avoid withdrawal. Jan is a good example:

Jan was so overwhelmed by her responsibilities at two different sites on her fieldwork experience, with two different supervisors, at a time when she had just broken up with her fiancé, that she called me to say that she didn't think she could continue. Jan cried throughout the conversation, frequently needing breaks to compose herself so that she could continue speaking. Jan needed time during the week to meet with a counselor she was seeing and to work on stress management.

After much talking and listening, it seemed to me that the experience would be doable if Jan could continue working part-time at only one site with one supervisor. I never get involved in communications between a student and his or her supervisor unless the student requests my help. In this case, Jan asked me to call to see if what we were requesting was possible. I agreed because I sensed that Jan was fragile and in a crisis stage. Also, the fieldwork coordinator with whom I schedule internships at Jan's fieldwork site was working at a different location from that of Jan. We both felt that something needed to be done immediately, and Jan did not think she would be able to reach the coordinator in the limited time she had between seeing patients. The fieldwork coordinator was quite understanding and agreed that Jan's two supervisors had very different styles and were probably putting a lot of stress on Jan to meet their individual requirements. She set up a part-time schedule with one of the supervisors, and the experience had a happy ending.

In another situation, a student's father and grandfather died within 1 week. The student was three-fourths of the way through her internship. She needed a leave of absence, not a withdrawal, and the facility was amenable to her doing that because she was a good student and all observations indicated that she would pass the internship. One other time that I intervened occurred when I withdrew a student from fieldwork after I received a phone call from an emergency room physician who had just met with my student because of suicidal ideation. The stress of the internship, being away from home, and ongoing depression were too much all at once. After the student received treatment, she went home, and I was able to reschedule her at an internship near her home where she had family and professional support.

Another occasion when withdrawal is requested occurs when a student has chosen to do an optional internship experience and then decides he or she would like to end earlier than originally planned. This is not an appropriate withdrawal. The facility has made a commitment of a specific time period to the student and has agreed not to take other students in order to give a good fieldwork experience to the student. When a student feels that he or she has already learned all he or she wants to learn, it says to the supervisor and others in the setting that what they are offering the student is not very good or not a learning experience. Making a commitment and then breaking it is unprofessional behavior.

If you are feeling overwhelmed at your internship, try this exercise. On one side of a piece of paper, list all the aspects of the internship that you feel are in control. These could be as simple as arriving to work on time or as significant as interacting well with the patients. On the other side of the page, list all those aspects that you feel are out of control or causing stress.

Examples of aspects of the internship in which they are not in control from previous students' experiences are difficulty completing the documentation on time, writing treatment plans with alternative activities for each goal for each patient every day, and cotreating with your supervisor. This list will help you to identify specific concerns and might help you, your supervisor, and your AFWC determine if there are ways to adapt the current situation to make it less stressful, or if it might be best to withdraw from the internship, work on areas of weakness, and begin again at a different site. Finally, if you are overwhelmed and feeling stress, identify those activities that help you to relieve stress, and work them into your day. One student who was working every spare minute to complete the paperwork requirements of an internship believed that she did not have any opportunity to take a walk or meditate. Her supervisor agreed to eliminate one of her daily treatment plans if she promised to use the time to do a stress-relieving activity. Within a week, she was handling all of her responsibilities better.

After the Withdrawal

If, after talking with significant others, your supervisor, and your AFWC, the decision is to withdraw from the experience, you need to follow your school's policies and procedures. Students are often required to create a remediation plan to present to the AFWC. The remediation plan must address issues of concern at the fieldwork, how the student plans to work on them, and what will make the next internship a successful one for the student. The list you made in thinking through your decision to withdraw will be helpful again. For each area that you felt was not in control, write a treatment plan for yourself. Add to the list anything that your supervisor listed as a concern. This can form the basis for your plan. The outcome should be how you and your AFWC will know that you have adequately addressed the area of concern and are ready for another fieldwork experience.

Meeting your own treatment goals should give you a sense of confidence as you begin again. Remember, you have made the best decision considering the time and the circumstances. Take the best that you can from the internship. Build on what you have learned, and move on.

If your withdrawal is due to personal reasons other than the internship, like personal illness or death of a family member, you need to take the time you need to get well or grieve. Keep your AFWC advised of your progress so that a new internship can be scheduled for you. You may need to be patient because internships are not always easy to find.

Students ask if what they have done at one setting can count toward another when they continue. The answer is, "No." Your supervisor must be able to certify at the end of your internship that you can function as an entry-level practitioner at that facility. To determine entry-level status, the supervisor needs to see the student progress through the learning stages toward functioning independently. Two shorter experiences would enable the student to reach midterm at two different places, not to function as an entry-level practitioner at one facility.

TERMINATIONS

Failing a course in school is not a pleasant experience. Failing an internship can be devastating because it is the equivalent of failing an entire semester of courses. If your fieldwork educator has been giving you feedback about your performance, termination should come as no surprise, but it can be devastating, nevertheless. I frequently describe a termination as a speed bump in the process of becoming an occupational therapy practitioner. Sometimes, the effect of having to slow down enables you to be more prepared for and to learn more from the next fieldwork experience.

Your AFWC should be aware of the situation and should be there to help you emotionally, as well as

technically, as you follow all of the facility's and school's policies and procedures for termination. Most contracts require that a facility let the school know if there are concerns about a student's ability to pass an internship. Hopefully, your supervisor shared his or her concerns with you, and you have been given a chance to respond to those concerns through a learning contract. If you were unable to meet the objectives of the learning contract by the deadline, termination is generally the outcome. You should understand that, if you are not able to meet the requirements for entry-level performance, judgment, or attitude by the end of the fieldwork experience, it is the obligation of the fieldwork educator to give you a failing grade or terminate your experience. The fieldwork educator is a gatekeeper to the profession with the responsibility of "...ensuring that the student is a safe, ethical, competent entry-level practitioner" (McCarron & Crist, 2000, p. 17). Occasionally, students are terminated without a learning contract because of safety or judgment issues that are considered too grave to allow the student to stay. Supervisors tell me that a student is terminated on the spot if a staff member would lose his or her job if he or she committed these same lapses in judgment or lack of safety precautions. Examples of such situations include confidential patient notes left in a common room for other patients or visitors to read, cabinets that are locked for patients' safety left unlocked, failure to use safety tools such as gait belts, and inappropriate physical contact with a patient.

Rogers and Elbert (2000) suggest some coping strategies for students who are being terminated that are relevant here. The first is learning from the experience. This includes developing a plan for the next internship. You should have a meeting with your supervisor in which he or she identifies the specific reasons for the termination as well as your positive contributions (McCarron & Crist, 2000). If you so desire, your AFWC can be present, either in person or by way of a conference phone call. When discussing the reasons for the termination, you should have the opportunity to respond to concerns of the facility. You should also ask any questions of clarification that will help you to see what you could have done differently. This is the first step toward learning from the experience. If your supervisor is not prepared to share strengths as well as weaknesses, you should ask. It is healthy to have a balanced view of yourself in the situation, so you can see what you have done well in addition to what you need to work on.

Second, Rogers and Elbert (2000) suggest that you vent appropriately. In the facility, you will be expected to handle yourself professionally. You can let others know of your disappointment. If you try to act as if you are unaffected by this experience, some will question whether you really understand the gravity of the situation. Hopefully, you will have a support group of family and/or friends who will listen to your feelings at length. Your AFWC will be happy to let you vent, but try to use your time talking to him or her efficiently; you will have many other details to discuss with him or her. In addition to talking to your support group, I recommend two very different activities that might help. One is some form of physical activity that you enjoy, and the other is journaling.

Third, "separate the person from the failure. You failed fieldwork. You are not a failure" (Rogers & Elbert, 2000, p. 14). It is very easy to say as one student said to me, "Okay, so I can't do it, and I'll never be an occupational therapy practitioner. I've wasted the past 4 years." Statements like these are unfair to you and are untrue. You are not a failure. You have had a failed experience, and it does not feel good, but it does not generalize to all areas of your life, to all areas of occupational therapy, or to all requirements of this internship. Get out that sheet on which you listed your strengths, and concentrate on the left-hand column, the one with the strengths. Visualize yourself doing those aspects of the internship in which you were successful. Now, you are ready to concentrate on working on those aspects of the internship in which you were unsuccessful. Concentrate on success.

Before you leave the facility, you should have the opportunity to provide feedback to the supervisor and others at the facility via your supervisor about your experience (McCarron & Crist, 2000). This assessment is based on your perceptions, but could be valuable as a learning experience for your supervisor in working with other students. If you feel you did not know soon enough that you were in trouble, mention it. If you felt that there was no time to learn or refine procedures before being expected to carry them out with patients, suggest how this could be handled differently. At all times, be professional. It is preferable to be able to talk about this with your supervisor, but sometimes students feel the best they can do is write comments on the student evaluation of fieldwork experience form.

After the Termination

You should have no contact with your fieldwork supervisor or others at the facility where you did your internship after a termination. All communication between you and the fieldwork site should be through your AFWC. If you want to appeal the termination, you will need to ask your AFWC about the procedure. Depending on the type of termination, the procedure may be different. There should be grievance committees, however, who will listen to your side of the story, look at documentation from the fieldwork site, and make a determination of whether or not your fieldwork should be labeled as a failure.

It is essential that you meet with your AFWC after a termination to go over the policies and procedures related to failing an internship and what you should do next. This initial meeting with the AFWC should not happen immediately. Students need time to settle feelings and be reflective of the experience. Often, a 1-week, or more, grieving period is needed before meeting with the AFWC. In most cases, you will probably not be allowed to continue with your fieldwork sequence until you have addressed the concerns of the fieldwork site. In some instances, failing an internship is equivalent to being terminated from the academic program; some schools terminate a student from the program after failing two internships. If you are in either of these categories, you will need to find out what your options are for switching to another major in the college or graduating with a degree without the internships.

THANK YOU NOTES

Once you have had some distance in time and space from the withdrawal or termination, it is a good idea to write a note to your supervisor and thank him or her for the part he or she has played in your learning experience. This provides closure for both of you. Maybe your supervisor was very supportive and sympathetic; maybe you knew how your supervisor agonized over the decision but knew that it would be best for you in the long run. Whatever the scenario, realize that no one likes to fail a student. Each and every supervisor I have talked with who had to terminate a student felt guilt and remorse. They all felt like they had failed in some way. A note to tell him or her what you have learned from the experience will help him or her to realize that there are no negative experiences, only learning experiences. Have your AFWC proofread your note before sending it to make sure your positive attitude is clear. Remember, the occupational therapy community is small, so it is important to reconstruct any burned bridges.

THE NEXT INTERNSHIP

Once you have met your learning objectives and your AFWC has found another internship site for you, you are ready to start again with your newfound knowledge and skills. Rules about student confidentiality preclude your AFWC from mentioning that you have failed or withdrawn from an internship unless you explicitly give your permission for him or her to do so. The question students frequently ask is, "What should I tell my next supervisor about my last experience?" Each person has to say what "fits" for him or her. I highly recommend, however, not trying to hide the experience. Eventually, it may slip out accidentally, and you will be more embarrassed than if you had been honest to begin with. If you have spent some time off between internships, you may be asked what you did during the past 6 months since your academic courses ended. I suggest that you say something like, "I had some difficulty on my last internship. This is what I learned..., and this is what I hope to continue working on. My strengths are...." Your AFWC can help you with the wording of this, but remember, you have to feel comfortable saying it. Students are frequently concerned that supervisors will think less of them if they say they did not complete an internship because they needed to practice some of their skills a little more. Quite contrary to this belief, most supervisors who have worked with students who are repeating internships have been very accepting and willing to work hard with the student on the major areas of concern.

SUPPORT FOR/FROM FRIENDS

I do hope that all students have support groups of peers while they are on their internships. The era of e-mail has made communication across distances much less time-consuming and costly, so students can keep in touch more easily. If you are providing support for a fellow student who is having difficulty and thinking about withdrawing from the fieldwork experience, please remind your friend to contact the AFWC for your school. If your friend is ill or dealing with a tough personal situation, remind him or her that there will be fieldwork placements at a later date and that your friend should work on his or her emotional/physical health so that he or she can be there for future patients/clients. If your friend is feeling like a total failure because of feedback from a supervisor and believes that he or she might be terminated, remind him or her to contact the AFWC and share these concerns. Let your friend vent and help him or her to see any learning experiences that are obvious to you. Remind your friend of all of the positive aspects of his or her personality and abilities.

If you are in need of support, call on one of your friends from school who may be currently on an internship and may be better able to empathize than anyone else.

SUMMARY

There will be some students from each program who will need to withdraw from an internship or who will be terminated from one. This chapter has provided information to help the student negotiate through what might be perceived as a very stressful time. While going through the experience of a withdrawal or termination, it will be next to impossible to think of it as a positive experience. However, after the fact, most students feel that it was a time of tremendous growth. With the help of the AFWC, the student should be able to create learning objectives and be a better occupational therapy practitioner in the end. The important vision to keep in mind is future success.

REFERENCES

Ilott, I. (1995). To fail or not to fail? A course for fieldwork educators. Am J Occup Ther, 49, 250-255.

Kyler-Hutchison, P. (1994, October 13). Fear of failure. OT Week. 256-257.

McCarron, K., & Crist, P. (2000). Supervision and mentoring. In S. Merrill & P. Crist (Eds.), Meeting the fieldwork challenge: A self-paced clinical course from AOTA. Bethesda, MD: The American Occupational Therapy Association, Inc.

Rogers, M. W., & Elbert, W. (2000). Measuring student fieldwork performance. In S. Merrill & P. Crist (Eds.), Meeting the fieldwork challenge: A self-paced clinical course from AOTA. Bethesda, MD: The American Occupational Therapy Association, Inc.

Section IV

TRANSITIONS

Chapter 13

TRANSITION MODELS

Sandy Bell, PhD, PT

Danielle slowly climbed the stairs to her third floor apartment. She was exhausted. Danielle had been at her final fieldwork site, St. Joseph's Community Hospital, for 3 weeks now, yet still had not adjusted to the 7:30 am starting time. She had never been a "morning person" and was now quite sure she could never become one. There was something else, too, she thought to herself as she closed the door behind her and hung up her coat. An unsettling feeling nagged at her, but she could not seem to put her finger on it. Her experience at St. Joseph's was going well. She liked the variety of patients and the freedom her supervisor gave her—too much freedom at times, she thought. Though Danielle did not feel she needed to work on cases with her supervisor, as she had in prior assignments, she wanted to. She was eager to collaborate more with her supervisor and the other team members. Among the day's mail was a letter from the director of a long-term care facility in her hometown. She had had an informational interview with him right before starting at St. Joseph's. It was a polite letter thanking her for her interest in the facility, with a regret that no openings were anticipated in the next 6 months. Danielle wondered how she would ever land her first job—so many facilities seemed to be in a hiring freeze. Though she had hoped to return to her hometown to start her career, she imagined she would have to move to another area of the country. The next piece of mail was the Visa bill—another $42 in interest this month, and she'd have to carry over a balance again. She was anxious to start working so she could pay in total her bills each month and start making payments on her school loan. There was a message on the machine from her boyfriend—he'd call her back later tonight. Over supper, Danielle made a detailed mental note of the treatment plan she had in mind for a patient she planned to see the next day. Her name was Lee Ann. She was 25 years old and just a few months older than Danielle. The more she worked with Lee Ann, the more Danielle liked her and cared about her as a person. Lee Ann had been beaten by her husband. She had sustained a closed head injury and had an array of physical and cognitive problems. Danielle abhorred the idea of domestic violence but had never met a victim of such abuse. When she thought of what happened to Lee Ann, she felt disturbed and angry inside. Danielle's thoughts shifted to her parents, who had divorced when she was 14 years old. There had been a lot of arguing, she remembered. Just then, the phone rang...

Danielle's story illustrates that fieldwork can be a time during which a student experiences many changes at personal and professional levels. From shifts in perceptions about intimacy and professional identity to relocating and attaining your first job, these types of changes can represent transitions, which are a fundamental part of adulthood. As an occupational therapy practitioner, you will experience change in some way on a constant basis. By its very nature, the course of patient therapy and rehabilitation is one of continual change—from one functional state (physical, cognitive, or emotional) to another. You will be an agent of change in your patients' lives and, by extension, in the lives of their family members and in their communities. Many of your patients will perceive you to be an integral part of a major transition in their lives.

At the same time, you will be experiencing your own life changes on personal and professional levels. Some changes will be directly related to the care you provide your patients; many will not. How you experience and adapt to transitions will be influenced by your perceptions of the changes associated with them. Your knowledge of concepts and processes involved in adult transitions may enhance your perceptions of changes you experience as well as choices you consider in adapting to the changes.

The purpose of this chapter is to provide an overview of the nature of adult transitions, illustrate how transition concepts and processes can be applied to individuals in clinical settings, and explore the types of transitions you may experience during fieldwork. Specifically, by the end of the chapter, you will be able to do the following:

➡ Describe key concepts and processes contained in leading adult transition models.

➡ Discuss strategies that can facilitate successful adaptation to changes associated with transition.

➡ Understand relationships between clinical reasoning style and perception of transition.

➡ Recognize types of transitions that are commonly experienced by students during fieldwork.

➡ Complete activities in which you apply your knowledge to enhance your awareness of factors associated with transitions during fieldwork.

TRANSITION MODELS

Life changes and transitions are such a fundamental part of adulthood that they have been studied by philosophers, psychologists, artists, and educators. Earlier researchers in this field focused on identifying transitions commonly experienced by adults in the United States at specific ages (Levinson, Darrow, Klein, Levinson, & McGee, 1978) or in specific stages of life (Lowenthal, Thurnher, & Chiriboga, 1975). More recently, however, researchers (Bridges, 1991; Schlossberg, Walters, & Goodman, 1995) have recognized the great variability in life experiences of American adults and have focused instead on describing processes that seem to be experienced by adults in transition regardless of age or life stage. One of the most frequently referenced models of adult transitions is Schlossberg's (1984, 1994) model of analyzing human adaptation to transition. Because of its wide application, this model will be used primarily as a framework for reviewing important concepts and processes associated with adult transitions.

Transition Beginnings

Schlossberg (1994), a practicing psychologist and a university professor, defines a *transition* as an event or nonevent that results in changes in assumptions about one's self and the world and subsequent changes in one's behavior and relationships. A transition is most often triggered by an event or something specific that happens (e.g., relocating to a new community). A transition can also be triggered by a nonevent or something specific that does not happen (e.g., not getting the job on which you had your heart set). This "trigger" event or nonevent assumes a special meaning for an individual and is the impetus for re-examining aspects of one's life (Schlossberg, 1984). Sometimes, an individual can easily identify what triggered a change in his or her perceptions (e.g., a traumatic accident or a political event). Other times, the trigger is elusive, and an individual may be only able to consciously pinpoint the start of a transition long after its beginning.

A second key concept about transitions identified by Schlossberg (1984) is that "a transition is not so much a matter of change as of the individual's *perception* of change. A transition is a transition if it is so defined by the person experiencing it" (p. 7). For example, one student may feel not at all affected by a change in supervisors halfway into a fieldwork assignment, whereas another student may perceive the change as triggering a fundamental shift in the course of his or her professional development.

Bridges (1980), another scholar in adult transitions, stresses that the impact of a transition on one's life does not necessarily correspond to the apparent importance of the triggering event. What may seem to others and to you, at first, a relatively unremarkable

MARCO'S STORY

I have been an OT practitioner for 10 years now. I have worked with children and their families in school or home settings for most of that time. Four years ago, I moved from Phoenix to Las Cruces, N.M., so that I could work in the rural farming communities there. Most of the parents of these kids work as migrant farm laborers. Many families speak only Spanish in the home, and most have no health insurance. Many of the children with developmental disabilities have medical problems that have been neglected for years. I work with the children and their teachers in the school, but I need to work with the families so that there is follow-through. Often, I end up teaching an older sibling how to do the positioning and daily stretching because both parents work long hours. I work 4 days a week. On Friday evenings and Saturday mornings, I volunteer at the Adult Literacy Center in town teaching English as a second language.

If you had asked me when I was an OT student if I ever thought I'd be working with kids for most of my career, I would have told you, "no way." I had wanted to specialize in industrial occupational therapy, analyzing jobs and figuring out how to prevent injuries. In fact, I was rather disappointed when I was assigned to work in a rural school system in southern Texas for my final fieldwork experience. One day, my supervisor and I visited the home of one of the children. Both his hands and arms had been badly burned in an accident and needed daily ranging and splinting. The parents were illegal immigrants from Mexico. An extended family of 12 aunts, uncles, and cousins all lived in a little three-room, run-down house with no plumbing. I had never seen such poverty. Neither my supervisor, who was new to the area, nor I spoke Spanish, and no one at the home spoke English. We had asked for an interpreter, but she did not show. Everyone wanted to help with caring for Miguel, but we could not communicate. On the way back to school, I could tell my supervisor was very upset and frustrated. At the time, I felt sorry for the family, but I had seen several unfamiliar things and some unpleasant things during that fieldwork experience. This experience was one of many. I know now that that incident stayed with me and has been a big influence on the decisions I have made in my career and my personal life. I decided to stay in the Southwest and work in rural areas with underprivileged children. I have read many books and articles on the plight of migrant farm laborers in this country. I have helped collect signatures to get the legislature to ensure that they get minimum wages. I took Spanish courses, and now I volunteer to teach English as a second language. Many of my students are parents of the children I see for therapy. I did not know it at the time, but that visit to Miguel's home when I was a student was the thing that pointed me down this path I have been on for the past 10 years and that I hope to continue for another 10 years.

event may in fact be the trigger for a series of profound changes in your values and behaviors. The story told by Marco (see *Marco's Story*) illustrates how what seemed like a relatively insignificant event when it occurred led to significant changes in Marco's views about his role in his community and the course of his professional career.

Whereas Schlossberg (1984, 1994) states that a life transition begins with a triggering event or non-event, other transition theorists specify that this trigger represents for an individual some sort of ending (Bridges, 1980) or farewell (Hudson, 1991). Bridges specifies that letting go of old values and connections is necessary in making room for new ones. The ending may be physical (e.g., impaired use of a limb after a cerebral vascular accident), or it may involve relationships (e.g., moving away from your family and friends to attend school). Some endings may be gradual and unplanned (e.g., loss of religious faith over many years), while other endings occur "right on schedule" (e.g., complet-

ing the last day of your last fieldwork assignment). Endings students experience during fieldwork may trigger a perceived transition, including the discharge or death of a patient with whom you had a close relationship, a change in clinical supervisors or rotation assignment, or the loss of department personnel due to downsizing layoffs (see *Reflection Activity* on p. 146).

Transition Characteristics

According to Schlossberg (1994), a transition can be characterized according to seven different yet interrelated factors: role change, emotional affect, source, timing, onset, duration, and degree of stress involved. Many transitions are characterized by a change in roles and responsibilities. Some transitions may involve a role gain, such as starting an academic program, taking a job, or getting married. Other transitions involve the loss of a role or set of responsibilities. Graduating from school, being laid off from

REFLECTION ACTIVITY

Take a few moments to reflect on your experiences in this fieldwork assignment or in a past assignment. Have any of your fieldwork experiences triggered a change in your values or assumptions related to any aspect of your preparation to be an occupational therapy practitioner? If yes, what were your values or assumptions before, and how have they changed? Have you changed your behavior because of these changes in your values and assumptions? Can you identify any specific event or nonevent that may have triggered this transition in your attitudes and behaviors?

your job, or moving away from home are examples of transitions in which role loss is a key factor. Often, the loss of one role leads to the gain of another. Relocating to a new community involves changes in old relationships and establishing new ones. The death of a parent after a long illness may mean ending your role as a primary caregiver and assuming responsibilities as head of the family.

A second characteristic of transitions is the emotions, or affect, you associate with it. Frequently, individuals associate positive feelings, such as joy and satisfaction, with life changes that involve gain or inclusion, such as a promotion with pay raise. Negative feelings, including guilt, sadness, or anxiety, are often associated with changes that involve loss or exclusion, such as the break up of a significant relationship.

The source of changes associated with a transition is a third factor that determines the nature of a transition (Schlossberg, 1994). The source can be internal (i.e., originating from personal volition). Choosing to take a year off after graduation before entering the workforce is an example of transition with an internal source. When changes associated with a transition originate from something other than personal volition, their source is external. Other people or specific circumstances may be the source of changes that seem forced upon an individual (Schlossberg, 1994). Taking a year off from school because you did not receive a scholarship, which was to be your primary source of financial support, is an example of a transition with an external source.

Three additional transition characteristics have to do with time. One factor describes the relative timing of a transition in the course of an individual's life. Though they may be largely unaware of it, most adults have built-in social clocks by which they judge a life event to be "off time" or "on time" (Schlossberg, 1994). A woman who returns to school at age 40 after her children have left home to complete a degree

in occupational therapy may perceive her transition into the profession to be off time. Certainly, she will be labeled as a "nontraditional" student by the educational institution. Entry into the profession by a "traditional-aged" student at the age of 25 will be perceived as on time and consistent with societal norms.

Pace of onset is another time-related factor that contributes to the nature of a transition. Some types of transitions are gradual, characterized by a series of subtle, often anticipated, changes over time. Graduation from an academic program and entry into the job market are examples of a transition with a gradual onset (Schlossberg, 1994). Other transitions have a sudden onset and are often unexpected. Contracting a serious long-term illness is an example of this type of transition.

The duration of changes associated with a transition also relate to time. Changes may be perceived as being permanent or temporary, or one can be uncertain of their duration. For example, when you start your first position employed as an occupational therapy practitioner, you may perceive it as a relatively short-term commitment in pursuit of your long-term career goals. After setting up your own private practice, however, you may expect that the change to self-employment is permanent. During times of economic uncertainty in the health care field, you may feel uncertain about the duration of any new professional position.

The final factor characterizing the nature of a transition is the degree of stress one associates with it. Some degree of physiological and psychological stress is associated with any transition, whether perceived as positive or negative, on time or off time, gradual or sudden (Schlossberg, 1994). If you perceive the stress as manageable, it can impel you to make decisions and to take action. Conversely, stress that is perceived as overwhelming can be an immobilizing force.

TRANSITION CHECKLIST

➠ Take your time.
➠ Do not act for the sake of acting.
➠ Arrange temporary structures.
➠ Take care of yourself in little ways.
➠ Get someone to talk to.
➠ Recognize that transition has a characteristic shape.

Adapted from Bridges, W. (1980). *Transitions*. Reading, MA: Addison-Wesley.

Transition Endings

Though the outcomes of a transition may have long-term effects in a variety of life contexts, the transitional episode itself is of limited duration. Adults may go through periods of relative stability in their lives, marking the end of transitions that previously dominated life experience. Whereas the beginning of a transition is often marked by a triggering event or nonevent, the end of a transition is often difficult to pinpoint. As you are the only one who can feel you are in transition, only you can feel that the transition has ended. Schlossberg (1994) posits that adaptation to a transition occurs when an individual is no longer preoccupied with it and has integrated the changes into his or her life. A conclusion is realized when an individual has assimilated the psychological and behavioral changes related to the transition. Marco's Story (p. 145) illustrates these concepts about transition endings. Marco describes changes in his values and assumptions regarding human rights and his role in serving his community triggered by a home visit experience he had during his final fieldwork assignment. These affective changes propelled him into making decisions that significantly impacted his career and personal life. Ten years after his visit to Miguel's home, Marco is now "living" those decisions and has fully integrated the emotional and behavioral changes triggered by that event.

Adaptation

Bridges (1980) refers to the time between the beginning and the ending of a transition as the "neutral zone" and what happens in the neutral zone as "a kind of street crossing procedure" (p. 112). For Schlossberg (1994), this is the period when adaptation to the changes associated with a transition occurs. Based on her work and that of her colleagues counseling adults in transition, Schlossberg found that individuals tend to have more difficulty adapting to transitions with certain types of characteristics. In general, an individual is more challenged when the changes associated with a transition evoke negative emotional feelings, are of an external source that is out of one's control, happen suddenly, are of uncertain duration, and occur at a time during which the individual is already experiencing high stress in his or her life. The process of adapting to changes associated with a transition can provide opportunities for personal growth, or, Schlossberg emphasizes, the process can present risk of psychological deterioration.

If you find yourself in a transition with many of the characteristics listed above, you may experience high stress for prolonged periods and be at risk for illness or exacerbation of pre-existing medical conditions (Holmes & Rahe, 1967). Bridges (1980) proposes using a "transition checklist" to facilitate coping with changes (see *Transition Checklist*). The first item on the transition checklist is a reminder to "take your time." While some situations may require your immediate response, many others can be observed and left to unfold at their own pace. This point is captured in a second checklist item: "Don't act for the sake of acting." A third item, "Arrange temporary structures," directs you to focus initially on setting up an environment in which your basic needs of shelter, food, and emotional supports are met. Balance this focus with efforts to "take care of yourself in little ways." Try to maintain a few treasured continuities in your life, such as a daily walk or a weekly movie. In addition, Bridges wisely prompts us to "get someone to talk to." Articulation of your thoughts and feelings is an extremely effective way to examine your beliefs and assumptions and the underlying reasons for the nature of your transition experience. The person to whom you talk, a professional or a friend, needs to be somewhat removed from your situation and nonjudgmental. The final item on Bridges' transition checklist is a cue to "recognize that transition has a characteristic shape," meaning that transitions tend to have a beginning, middle, and an end. Reminding yourself of the adage "nothing ever stays the same" or "this too shall pass" may help you to endure the stressful times.

Transition Models Summary

To review, transitions have a beginning, set off by some sort of trigger. The trigger may be or may not be directly related to the nature of the changes that follow it. Transitions are marked by changes in values and assumptions that lead to changes in the choices one makes and in one's behavior. Transitions can be relatively small and impact a few aspects of one's life, or they can be large and impact many aspects of life. Factors that affect the nature of a transition include role change (gain or loss), affect (positive or negative), source (internal or external), timing (on time or off time), onset (gradual or sudden), duration (permanent, temporary, or uncertain), and degree of stress. Using specific coping strategies may facilitate an individual's successful adaptation to the changes associated with a transition. The end of a transition is realized when an individual moves from being totally preoccupied with the transition to integrating the changes associated with it into his or her life.

Fieldwork and Transitions

You may apply your knowledge of the concepts and processes involved in adult transitions to enhance your fieldwork experiences in three ways: to recognize the effect clinical reasoning style can have on perception of transition, to be responsive to the experience of patients who find themselves in transition while in your care, and to successfully adapt to the life changes you will invariably experience as you transition from your final fieldwork assignment and graduation to your first year as an occupational therapy practitioner.

Transition Experience and Clinical Reasoning

In their seminal Clinical Reasoning Study, Mattingly and Fleming (1994) documented that occupational therapists use multiple forms of reasoning in fulfillment of professional responsibilities. They found that, in patient assessment and treatment, therapists use predominantly three forms of reasoning: *procedural*, *interactive*, and *conditional*. For this reason, Mattingly and Fleming describe therapists as having a "three-track mind."

Procedural Reasoning

Therapists use procedural reasoning when they identify and classify patient problems and select the most appropriate procedures to address those problems. This process often involves an analytical approach to problem solving. The first and perhaps most important step in the process is problem identification, which is largely dependent upon a therapist's perception of the patient's problem situation (Mattingly & Fleming, 1994). The attributes of a situation a therapist chooses to observe are largely dependent upon the therapist's level of experience with similar types of situations. Prior experience, in both professional and personal realms, becomes a "lens" through which a therapist perceives and assesses a patient problem. Experience influences the situational "cues" or "clues" to which a therapist will attend, how the therapist perceives interrelationships among those cues and prior knowledge stored in memory, and ultimately the decisions the therapist makes regarding therapeutic procedures.

Interactive Reasoning

Whereas procedural reasoning requires interacting and establishing rapport with patients to make observations and test hypotheses regarding the effectiveness of therapeutic strategies, this mode of reasoning is largely noninteractive, relying on the therapist's own cognitive processes. Interactive reasoning, the second form of reasoning employed by occupational therapists, however, is entirely dependent upon interactions between therapist and patient. Interactive reasoning focuses on facilitating the patient's commitment to the therapeutic process. Mattingly and Fleming (1994) define *interactive reasoning* as a therapist's "therapeutic use of self," characterized by working collaboratively with the patient as a partner in the therapeutic process. Through reasoned interactions with the patient and with other essential members of the patient's world, a therapist seeks to appreciate patient perspectives and values, to establish goals that are meaningful for the patient, and to motivate the patient to achieve those goals. Interactive reasoning requires the ability to be consciously aware of how one's own perspectives and motives enter into the therapeutic process and to ensure that the process remains collaborative at all times. On occasion, a therapist may choose to interact with a patient in ways that fall outside of boundaries defined by procedural reasoning processes. The sharing of personal life stories and the exchanging of gifts with a patient are examples of this type of interactive behavior.

YOUR CLINICAL REASONING STYLE

Take a moment to reflect on the following questions related to your style of clinical reasoning:
➡ What do you perceive to be your primary role as an occupational therapy practitioner?
➡ Is your role linked to a clinical reasoning style?
➡ Do you have a predominant style? Is it more procedural, interactive, or conditional? Or is it a combination of styles?

Conditional Reasoning

The final track in the occupational therapist's three-track mind is that of conditional reasoning. This type of reasoning is directed toward understanding the patient as a "whole person"—an individual with a past, present, and future. It seeks to understand how the patient's experience of impaired function and disability fit into the conditions or context of his or her life-world (Mattingly & Fleming, 1994). Whereas interactive reasoning focuses on a therapist's therapeutic use of self as a means of collaborating with the patient to meet relatively short-term goals, conditional reasoning focuses on enabling the patient to construct a meaningful future life-world of which the therapist is no longer an integral part. The expression of conditional reasoning is the construction of meaningful and meaning-making experiences with the patient directed toward the realization of his or her future life. In this type of reasoning, a therapist uses imagination and symbolism in order to create experiences with the patient that offer choice in activities and motives. By choosing between courses of action, the patient develops intentionality in focusing his or her energy, which is critical to actualizing life goals (Mattingly & Fleming, 1994).

Individual Differences in Clinical Reasoning

Mattingly and Fleming (1994) found that two factors, level of experience and personal style, had the strongest impact on the ways in which occupational therapists developed and used clinical reasoning skills. Novice therapists tend to view their role as completing evaluation and treatment procedures. They cultivate procedural reasoning skills directed toward classifying a patient's clinical condition and selecting the most appropriate procedures to address the condition. Novices may also be preoccupied with developing their interactive reasoning skills and may devote much concern to establishing rapport with patients. Novice therapists tend to develop conditional-reasoning abilities last because abilities in the other two domains may be prerequisites to understanding the more global phenomenon of the patient's life experience. In addition, novices tend to compartmentalize their knowledge and vacillate their attention back and forth between the various modes of reasoning, particularly between the procedural and interactive modes (Mattingly & Fleming, 1994).

More experienced therapists tend to have well-developed reasoning skills in each domain. They are able to use the skills simultaneously in an integrative fashion, changing emphasis from one domain to the other as indicated (Mattingly & Fleming, 1994). The knowledge base of seasoned therapists can have great breadth and depth, with many interconnections across domains. It includes knowledge gained from personal as well as professional experiences. Whereas novices tend to approach clinical problem solving by finding the right answers to solve the problem, therapists who are more proficient focus on assessing the situation to find the right questions.

Though these generalizations about clinical reasoning characteristics between novice and experienced occupational therapists have held true across a variety of clinical settings, Mattingly and Fleming (1994) observed that therapists tend to develop a clinical reasoning "style" or preference for using one reasoning mode over the other two, regardless of level of experience (see *Your Clinical Reasoning Style*). Predominant reasoning style is influenced largely by a therapist's professional values and role perception. Some therapists view their role as addressing procedural concerns. They tend to focus on the functions of the physical body and may view personal interaction as peripheral to meeting treatment goals. Other therapists strongly value establishing an interactive relationship with their patients, where the relationship itself becomes a therapeutic tool. They may address concerns of self-image and social functioning more than physical functioning. A third group of therapists have well-developed conditional reasoning skills. They place most value on their role in facilitating the patient's construction of a meaningful future.

Clinical Reasoning Style and Transition Experience

Your fieldwork assignments require you to change your learning environment from academic classroom to clinical workplace. They may also involve your moving to a new community on a temporary basis, being away from significant others, and increasing the demand on your financial resources. Fieldwork also necessitates changing your daily routine, assuming new roles and responsibilities, establishing many new relationships in a relatively short period, and maintaining close contact with injured or ill individuals, many of whom are in the midst of major life transitions. Subsequently, fieldwork is often a period when students find themselves in transition. At a time when you are focused on developing your clinical reasoning skills, you may find that an experience related to providing patient care has impacted you to the extent that you feel core values and assumptions are shaken, old ways of behaving are inadequate, and you are unsure of how to behave in the future.

Your style of clinical reasoning, whether predominantly procedural, interactive, or conditional, will influence largely what you attend to, or "pay attention to," when working with patients. The same event may have a different impact on you depending upon your clinical focus at the time. For example, your experience of the death of a very ill older patient whom you cared deeply about at a time when you are focused on interactive reasoning may trigger a transition for you in terms of valuing and maintaining important relationships. You may reach a new appreciation of the potential frailty of life and subsequently enhance your relationship with your elderly parents through sharing more life activities with them. This same event may have a different meaning for you if it occurs when you are immersed in procedural aspects of care. It may trigger feelings of inadequacy in your abilities to make effective choices for care and questioning whether you have chosen a profession in which you can excel as a clinician. You may choose to discuss the unsettling feelings with someone you trust. Last, if the lens through which you perceived this event was opened wide to the conditional elements of your role as a therapist, you may experience a transformation in your understanding for the multitude of factors that affect health and quality of life. The transition for you may involve modifying your own self-care habits, such as making a commitment to meditate on a daily basis and exercising more regularly.

UNDERSTANDING PATIENT TRANSITIONS

In the previous section, you explored how your approach to clinical reasoning can influence your perception of how key clinical experiences impact your values, assumptions, and behaviors. The values, assumptions, and behaviors of patients, too, can be profoundly affected by how they perceive changes in their lives associated with their clinical condition and care. You can apply your knowledge of adult transitions to enhance your understanding of the meaning patients make of their changing life-world.

You will invite each patient to make a commitment to actively participate in the course of care and to make choices that give meaning to therapeutic activities. Appreciate that a patient's expression of intentionality in choice may be difficult if the patient is unsure of his or her future. Challenge yourself to develop your conditional reasoning skills in exploring future possibilities with the patient. The more you appreciate the various conditions of the patient's life-world, the better you can anticipate and adapt to the impact they may have on the patient's experience of the therapeutic process. By offering responsive care, you can best support the patient in transition.

Transition from Academic to Professional Life

This chapter began with a story about Danielle, a young woman in her final fieldwork assignment preparing to start her career as an occupational therapy practitioner. Her transition from student to new practitioner is filled with changes in her values and expectations regarding professional as well as personal aspects of her life. As a member of a health care team, Danielle is beginning to value collaboration and interdependence over independence in practice. In working with a particular patient, she is challenged to find a balance between objectivity and subjectivity and to use all three types of clinical reasoning—procedural, interactive, and conditional. Danielle is uncertain about her employment prospects and the ways in which changes in the nation's health care system will affect her chosen profession. Additionally, she does not know if she will need to relocate to another part of the country, and she is anxious over her financial situation. In the midst of these changes associated with the transition from student to new practitioner,

Danielle is experiencing another set of changes at a deep personal level. She is having strong emotional reactions to her new appreciation for the realities of domestic violence and she is finding links to her own family situation. Perhaps in the future, Danielle will perceive that her work with a victim of domestic violence during her final fieldwork experience triggered long-lasting changes in her values and life choices.

Your knowledge of factors that characterize transitions can be used to assess in more detail the nature of Danielle's transition from student to new practitioner. The transition involves losing the role of student and gaining the role of licensed practitioner. Danielle has both positive and negative feelings associated with the changes she is experiencing. For example, she feels positive about her fieldwork experience, yet anxious about finances and finding her first job. Some of the changes, such as an effort to be more collaborative in practice, have been initiated internally. Other changes, such as the job market for new occupational therapy practitioners, have an external source and are out of her control. The overall timing of this transition in Danielle's life is consistent with that of societal expectations. The pace of the transition from student to new practitioner is gradual, marked by anticipated events including graduation, successful completion of the licensure exam, and the start of a new position. Some of the changes associated with Danielle's transition will be permanent, such as earning her degree. Other conditions she perceives as temporary in duration (e.g., her financial deficit). Uncertainty shrouds some aspects of the transition. For example, Danielle is uncertain about how long she will be unemployed after graduation.

Danielle is likely to feel challenged by many aspects of her transition. These aspects evoke negative feelings, are out of her control, or are of uncertain duration. Knowing what the challenges are will better prepare Danielle to cope with the negative stress that accompanies them. Other aspects of her transition, such as successful graduation and getting her first paycheck, may have an energizing effect. Danielle's successful adaptation to the changes associated with her transition from student to new practitioner will depend largely on her ability to recognize that new beginnings start with being open to new possibilities, releasing old assumptions, and being willing to try new behaviors.

The activities in *Transition Activities* (p. 152) provide you with an opportunity to apply your knowledge of concepts and processes involved in adult transitions to enhance your awareness of transitions you may experience during your own fieldwork. You can use this increased awareness as a first step in understanding how you tend to perceive changes associated with a transition, as well as how you consider choices in adapting to changes.

SUMMARY

In closing, as you complete the activities in *Transition Activities*, keep in mind the following nine points addressed in adult transition models:

➠ Transitions are a fundamental part of adulthood.

➠ A transition is characterized by a change in values and assumptions that leads to changes in choices and behaviors.

➠ Many transitions start with a trigger event or nonevent.

➠ A transition can be relatively small and impact a few aspects of life, or it can be large and impact many aspects of life.

➠ Successful adaptation to changes associated with a transition is more challenging if the changes evoke negative feelings, have an external source, happen suddenly, are of uncertain duration, and occur at a time when an individual is already experiencing high stress.

➠ The process of adapting to changes associated with a transition can provide opportunities for personal growth or present risk of psychological deterioration.

➠ The end of a transition is reached when an individual is no longer preoccupied with the changes associated with it and has assimilated them into his or her life.

➠ The transition from student to new practitioner can affect many personal and professional aspects of an individual's life.

➠ In the clinical setting, a practitioner's clinical reasoning style can influence how he or she perceives the impact of a trigger event and subsequent changes in attitudes and behaviors.

REFERENCES

Bridges, W. (1980). *Transitions*. Reading, MA: Addison-Wesley.

Bridges, W. (1991). *Managing transitions: Making the most of change*. Reading, MA: Addison-Wesley.

TRANSITION ACTIVITIES

In this activity, you will apply your knowledge of transition concepts and processes to enhance your awareness of transitions you may experience during your own fieldwork. Complete this activity during the second half of your fieldwork assignment. The activity is intended as a personal reflection, yet you may find that you would like to review your thoughts with your supervisor after completing the activity. On a separate sheet of paper, write your responses to each item. Do not concern yourself with grammar or spelling—getting your thoughts on paper is most important. Give yourself between 45 and 60 minutes to complete the activity.

1. First, make a list of the many life roles you are currently fulfilling (e.g., daughter or son, student therapist, friend, sibling, peer mentor, roommate, club member, etc.).
2. In what ways has fulfillment of your role as a student therapist on fieldwork assignment impacted your other life roles?
3. Have the changes in your other life roles:
   a. involved loss or gain in responsibilities?
   b. been accompanied by positive or negative emotions?
   c. been initiated by you or by something external?
   d. felt socially on time or off time?
   e. been gradual or sudden?
   f. been long-term, short-term, or of unknown duration?
   g. felt manageable or overwhelming?
4. In what ways have your perceptions (eg, assumptions, values, attitudes, or expectations) about your role as an occupational therapy practitioner changed over the course of this current fieldwork experience?
5. Describe a particular experience during this fieldwork assignment (or a past assignment) that you feel triggered changes in your perceptions about your role as an occupational therapy practitioner.
6. Because of the changes in your perceptions you described in question 4, in what ways have you modified your behaviors or the ways you make decisions as a student?
7. In what ways have the changes in your perceptions about your role as occupational therapy practitioner influenced your behaviors or ways you make decisions in personal aspects of your life?
8. Last, list three actions you could take if the stress associated with the changes you have experienced begins to feel overwhelming.

Holmes, T. H., & Rahe, R. H. (1967). The social readjustment rating scale. *J Psychosom Res, 2,* 213-218.

Hudson, F. M. (1991). *The adult years: Mastering the art of self-renewal.* San Francisco, CA: Jossey-Bass.

Levinson, D. J., Darrow, C. N., Klein, E. B., Levinson, M. G., & McGee, B. (1978). *The seasons of a man's life.* New York, NY: Knopf.

Lowenthal, M. F., Thurnher, M., & Chiriboga, D. (1975). *Four stages of life: A comparative study of women and men facing transitions.* San Francisco, CA: Jossey-Bass.

Mattingly, C., & Fleming, M. H. (1994). *Clinical reasoning: Forms of inquiry in a therapeutic practice.* Philadelphia, PA: F. A. Davis.

Schlossberg, N. K. (1984). *Counseling adults in transition.* New York, NY: Springer.

Schlossberg, N. K. (1994). A model for analyzing human adaptation to transition. *The Counseling Psychologist, 9*(2), 2-18.

Schlossberg, N. K., Walters, E. B., & Goodman, J. (1995). *Counseling adults in transition* (2nd ed.). New York, NY: Springer.

Chapter 14

Studying for the NBCOT Exam During Fieldwork

Karen Sladyk, PhD, OTR, FAOTA

As you are beginning or completing level II fieldwork, it is time to begin thinking about the certification exam for occupational therapists (OTs) or occupational therapy assistants (OTAs). The National Board for Certification in Occupational Therapy (NBCOT) is a private, nonprofit agency responsible for the development and administration of the certification exam for occupational therapists, registered (OTRs) and certified occupational therapy assistants (COTAs). Although a few work sites may not require certification, most governmental, regulatory, insurance, and other agencies use NBCOT examinations as a credentialing standard. Many states' licensing boards require passing the certification exam as the minimum standard for employment. The bottom line is that you must pass the appropriate NBCOT exam to initially practice occupational therapy.

This chapter is designed to help you understand the following by the end:

➡ The importance of an individualized study plan developed early in level II fieldwork.

➡ The basic certification process.

➡ Suggested study techniques and fieldwork review effective for certification exam success.

The program director at your school likely has already informed you about how to become eligible to sit for the examination. Students can stay up-to-date on the latest NBCOT policies and procedures by regularly checking www.nbcot.org. It is extremely important that students completely follow NBCOT's rules, as there are no exceptions to the rules. Students who make one error in the application process will be rolled over to the next certification exam date, thereby losing time. Beginning in 2003, NBCOT plans to have "on demand" testing opportunities.

OT and OTA
Examination Structure

Each exam has 200 multiple-choice questions. Each question has four possible answer choices labeled A, B, C, and D. There are no "all of the above" or combination choices on the OT or OTA exam. The questions are different on the OT and OTA exams, and the test bank is never mixed. The penalty for leaving an answer blank is the same as an incorrect answer, so be sure to fill in your best guess for all items. Choose only one answer for each question and key in your answer on the computer.

The examinations will be scored by the testing agency and then reviewed by an OT committee to look for flawed questions. After flawed questions are removed, criterion-referenced scoring will be used to calculate the passing score. This means that those people above the criterion score will pass the certification examination and those below will not. Your score is not compared to other people who took the exam, but simply to the minimum passing level to be an entry-level occupational therapy practitioner.

Test takers who need special accommodations due to a disability (such as visual, hearing, health, or orthopedic impairment; or learning, emotional, or multiple disabilities) will be provided with services as outlined in the Americans with Disabilities Act. Information on special accommodations is located in the candidate's handbook from NBCOT. It is important that you provide the documentation necessary and follow the specific process in the handbook.

Studying Ideas

Now that you understand basic NBCOT and certification process information, it is time to begin to make your study plan so you can be successful on the certification exam. You have had numerous past experiences studying for exams but this one is especially important because of the financial and personal costs. The integrative nature of this exam makes some college studying techniques, such as cramming, ineffective. Let's briefly review some studying ideas you may find helpful.

Study Groups

Studying a large amount of material with a group of people can be easier and more efficient. However, as you know, not all study groups are effective. You may have experienced a group project in school in which one or more participants did not do their fair share. This often leads to resentment and hurt feelings. If you plan to form a study group, ask people who you know will actively participate. If you are asked to join a study group, be sure you have a clear understanding of the group's goals and expectations. In any case, be sure to allow some time at the beginning of the first session to allow everyone an opportunity to share goals and expectations. If someone feels that he or she cannot participate, allow him or her to decline with dignity.

Exam Review Conferences

Many occupational therapy schools offer a 1- or 2-day conference to review content for the exam. You can call the American Occupational Therapy Association (AOTA) (if you are a member) or area occupational therapy schools to see if one is available. There are several for-profit businesses that also offer exam review programs. Check occupational therapy trade magazines such as *OT Advance* or *OT Practice* for educational listings.

Lecture Notes

Even though you may have had one class that you did not like, the faculty at your school provided you with a global education in occupational therapy. AOTA requires all occupational therapy programs to meet minimum standards to receive or maintain the school's accreditation. Your occupational therapy program has met the standard components. This means that your classes provided you with at least the minimum information needed to pass the exam. With all of that said, you should have everything you need to know about occupational therapy written down in your class lecture notes. Reviewing your notes is one of the most effective ways to study for the certification exam.

Textbooks

It would be impossible (and I do not recommend that you try) to reread your textbooks from cover to cover. Even if you did not sell them back to the bookstore for some extra cash, reading your textbooks in their entirety is not an effective use of study time.

It is appropriate to read your textbooks in the areas in which you are weak. I recommend that you read only the textbook sections in which you need detailed review. Use your notes from class to provide a basic study outline, and refer to the textbooks for more detail. Be sure to save your textbooks for your professional needs after the exam.

Specific Content Textbooks

Several books are available to make reviewing content more organized than reviewing textbooks from school. Outline books such as Reed's *Quick Reference to OT* (2000) and Sladyk's *OT Study Cards in a Box* (1999) can be helpful for review. Moyers (1999) wrote an excellent booklet that outlines the practice of occupational therapy in a concise manner. *The Guide to Occupational Therapy Practice* includes the most important position papers of the profession including Uniform Terminology and the Standards of Practice. The guide also presents a wonderful review of terminology, OT process with case examples, and ICIDH-2 perspectives. The guide can be purchased from the AOTA.

NBCOT Practice Test

NBCOT offers a practice test given by computer at local testing centers. This test is made up of 100 sample questions scored by the computer in the same format as the NBCOT exam. Currently, the computer does not provide information beyond the total number wrong. See the candidate's handbook for fees and application process.

Exam Style Study Question Books

Study question manuals present content in the form of multiple-choice questions. The questions are not practice or real questions from the exam but are study questions designed to help the student prepare for the exam. Several examples are reviewed in *Study Question Manual Review* (p. 158).

Author Bias

I am also an author of one of the study question manuals mentioned below as well as the study cards mentioned above. I believe the study question manuals available on the market are written by talented occupational therapy practitioners. I feel strongly that all can help you prepare for the NBCOT exam. Each study question manual provides a different approach. As the reader, you can select the best approach for you. The review on the next page is provided to help you choose the manual(s) that is right for you. The listing is in alphabetical order of title and was updated as of January 2002.

In addition to the above-mentioned books, Cottrell (2001) has published an exam review book included in International Educational Resources' exam review workshop. This content and study question book can be purchased independently. Costs of the exam review manuals range from $25 to $65.

ROLE OF FIELDWORK IN PREPARING FOR THE EXAM

The purpose of fieldwork is to integrate classroom study with clinical practice and to develop clinical reasoning skills. Much of what you know as an occupational therapy student was developed and refined during your fieldwork experiences. This section of the book is designed to help you use your fieldwork experience as you study for the exam. Opportunities to reflect on your areas of accomplishment and those that need further review before you take the exam are provided. Begin by reviewing all your level I and II fieldwork experiences. There are several ways to categorize your fieldwork experiences, but students often find it easiest to review their experience by diagnoses and by Uniform Terminology (AOTA, 1994) or the Practice Framework (pending RA approval in 2002). *Fieldwork Diagnosis Review* (p. 159) has diagnostic categories with which many OT practitioners work. It is not expected that you have had experiences in all these areas. On the contrary, students who focused their experiences in limited areas develop clinical reasoning skills more easily (Sladyk & Sheckley, 2000). This table is designed to point out which areas you are accomplished in and which areas may need more study for the exam. Use a check mark to indicate your assessment of your fieldwork experience. Blank spaces are provided at the end of the table to add other diagnostic categories.

After you have completed a review of your fieldwork experiences, it is time to make an assessment of the areas you need to review before the exam. Fieldwork was never intended to provide you with a view of all occupational therapy practice. Setting studying priorities for the exam should begin in the *no experience* and *observation experience* columns. Even with that as a starting place, you may feel like it is too much to manage at once. Use *Setting Study Priorities* (p. 160) to set your study priorities.

It may also be helpful to review your fieldwork experiences using the outline of Uniform Terminology (AOTA, 1994). Uniform Terminology is used in the NBCOT exam, and even with the current revision planning by AOTA, this document can be helpful in studying. *The Occupational Therapy Practice Framework* (AOTA, 2001) is expected to be presented to the Representative Assembly of AOTA at their spring 2002 voting meeting. Even if the framework

STUDY QUESTION MANUAL REVIEW

Title	Authors	Publisher	# of Questions	Year of Publication	Features
Examination Review: Occupational Therapy	Dundon	Appleton & Lange	800	1988 (has not been updated)	One page of support text. Four hundred non-OT questions to review sciences, 400 OT questions clustered in topic groups.
The Occupational Therapy Examination Review Guide (both OT and OTA versions available)	Johnson, Lurch, & DeAngelis	F. A. Davis	800 plus repeating 200	2001	Nine pages of support text. Four tests clustered in pediatrics, psychosocial, physical disability, and administration. A fifth test of repeating questions is mixed like the NBCOT exam.
OT Exam Review Manual (both OT and OTA versions are available)	Sladyk	SLACK Incorporated	500 to 550	2001	Thirty-three pages of support text. All questions are mixed like the NBCOT exam. Content and domain style questions. Includes chapters on study plans, fieldwork, life after the exam.
Study Guide for the OT Certification Examination (both OT and OTA versions available)	NBCOT	NBCOT	70	1999	Nineteen pages of support text. All questions are mixed like NBCOT exam.

replaces Uniform Terminology, the content of the current document is expected to be absorbed in the new framework. Use *Fieldwork Uniform Terminology Review* (p. 160) to review your fieldwork experiences, and then return to *Setting Study Priorities* to update your study priorities.

MAKING A STUDY PLAN

Several studying ideas were presented. Fieldwork students should begin to map out a plan early in their first level II fieldwork because balancing fieldwork expectations and exam studying might be a challenge. Some students may think that waiting until field-

FIELDWORK DIAGNOSIS REVIEW

Diagnosis	No Experience	Observation Experience	Some Experience	A Lot of Experience
AIDS				
Amputation				
Arthritis				
Bipolar disorder				
Burns				
Cancer				
Cardiac disease				
Cerebral palsy				
Child/elder abuse				
Cerebrovascular accident (CVA)				
Dementia				
Depression				
Drug/alcohol abuse				
Eating disorders				
Failure to thrive				
Hand/arm conditions				
Head injuries				
Kidney disease				
Learning disabilities/Attention deficit hyperactivity disorder (ADHD)				
Mental retardation/Pervasive developmental disorder (PDD)				
Multiple sclerosis				
Muscular dystrophy				
Orthopedic conditions				
Personality disorders				
Schizophrenia				
Sensory integration (SI) dysfunction				
Spina bifida				
Spinal cord injuries				
Wellness				

SETTING STUDY PRIORITIES

Top Priorities	*Plan of Action*
1.	1.
2.	2.
3.	3.
4.	4.
5.	5.
6.	6.

FIELDWORK UNIFORM TERMINOLOGY REVIEW

Performance Areas, Components, and Contexts	*No Experience*	*Observation Experience*	*Some Experience*	*A lot of Experience*
Activities of daily living (ADLs): grooming, dressing, eating, basic self-care				
Instrumental activities of daily living (IADLs): community skills, advanced self-care				
Home management				
Care of others				
Educational activities				
Vocational activities				
Play or leisure				
Sensory processing				
Perceptual processing				
Neuromusculoskeletal issues				
Motor issues				
Cognitive issues				
Psychosocial issues				
Temporal contexts: age, development, life stage, disability				
Environmental contexts: physical, social, culture				

Adapted from American Occupational Therapy Association. (1994). Uniform Terminology for occupational therapy. *Am J Occup Ther, 48*(11), 1047-1059.

work is done to begin studying is the best plan, but these students miss opportunities to discuss clinical problems with fieldwork educators during supervision.

Consider the story of Juan, completing a physical rehabilitation placement in Florida. Juan specifically planned this fieldwork after discussion with his academic fieldwork coordinator (AFWC) because he wanted experience with older adults with neurological and orthopedic issues. He was willing to temporarily move to a new state to get this experience because he felt neurological cases were a weakness for him. Unfortunately for his experience, the current caseload has very few neurologically involved occupational therapy consumers. However, Juan has been reviewing his textbooks and asking his supervisor about the case studies he has in his books. By initiating conversations such as, "What would you do if you had a client like..." Juan is experiencing his supervisor's clinical reasoning. These informal conversations allow Juan to take home extra experiences when he returns to his home state and prepares for the exam.

Now that you have set your study priorities (see *Setting Study Priorities* on p. 160), consider the amount of time available before the exam and what time you have outside of your current life demands. The exam is now offered four times per year with 3-week "windows of testing appointments." This means that exam opportunities are generally available within 3 months from when you are eligible. NBCOT plans to begin "on demand" testing sometime in 2003. Keep in mind the exams are computerized, and allow 4 hours to complete the 200-question test. Students do not know their results until about 3 weeks from the last appointment day. If you do not pass the exam the first time, restudy time is limited. What to do first is often a challenge for those beginning the exam studying process. *What To Do First* (p. 162) offers some suggestions.

COUNTDOWN CALENDAR

A blank calendar (see *Countdown Calendar* on p. 163) is provided to help you organize your last month before the exam. Use this calendar to chart your goals and study plans. Begin by entering the month and year you will take the exam. Enter the dates in each box. Mark your exam appointment at the testing center. Copy the calendar from the book and post it in a prominent place. Once you have a dated calendar for your goals, you can begin to develop your study plans.

PROBLEMS THAT INTERFERE WITH STUDYING

When Two Sources Disagree

A student wrote me once asking for my opinion about a specific question in *OT Exam Review Manual* where my information disagreed with the information she had been presented from another resource. I was happy to comment on this because, in an exciting and always changing profession like occupational therapy, there are times when different professionals disagree about an issue. My questions are study questions, designed to help you study for the exam. Because the questions are not exam questions, you may find a question where the answer disagrees with something you learned somewhere else. In the NBCOT exam, numerous people review each question, and exam authors use several references to check questions. Remember that NBCOT also removes any question from the exam after it has been administered if the question is found to be faulty. When faced with different information from two sources, use your best clinical judgment.

Motivation

Sometimes, it seems impossible to just sit down and study. Even if you do not have other things on your mind, there are a hundred other fun things to do than study for the certification exam. If this is happening to you, set very small goals. Begin with, I will study for 10 minutes, or I will complete five questions in a study question manual. When done, see if you can do it again. Keep rewards reachable, and encourage others not to sabotage your plans.

Use dead time in your schedule. For example, read content outlines or homemade flash cards while waiting for the bus, appointments, or for lunch. Even time in the elevator can be used to review a card. Post these cards in places where you can do two things at once such as drying your hair, cooking supper, or brushing your teeth. Find ways to make every minute count so that when you sit down for "official" study time, you already have made progress.

Test Anxiety

As you may remember in a psychopathology class you had years ago, anxiety rears its head in many ways. Indifference, guilt, anger, blame, and sadness all are symptoms of test anxiety (Ellis, 2000). Overcoming

WHAT TO DO FIRST

Time left to your exam	*Start your plan here*
6 or more months	Good for you; you have plenty of time to study. Decide what study guides or other books will provide you with the "just right challenge" and best support. Order these books. Map out a basic study plan; invite others to participate if appropriate. Visit the NBCOT web site. When books arrive, review, and begin studying 1 to 2 hours per week.
4 to 5 months	You planned well. Set study priorities. Read supporting information in study guides, begin content reviews using outlines from books. Formulate "what if" questions for fieldwork supervisor. Visit the NBCOT web site. Study 2 to 4 hours per week.
2 to 3 months	No need to panic; you have some time but you must be efficient. Visit the NBCOT web site. Make a serious study plan. Aim for an hour per day until the study guides and content books are complete, then adjust your study time from there.
About a month	Time to get serious. Scan above suggestions for ideas that work best for you. Aim for at least 1 to 2 hours of study per day, keeping a list of weak areas. Adjust plan from there.
2 to 3 weeks	If you ordered study question manuals, skip content chapters for now. Begin with questions, keeping a list of weak areas. Adjust your study plan from there. If you did not order study question manuals, review content using outline books mentioned above or review class notes. Aim for 2 to 4 hours of study per day.
Retesting	You are not alone, as 15% to 20% of candidates do not pass the exam the first time. Analyze with your AFWC or other professor what went wrong. Review possible study techniques to be added to your plan. Use campus services available to you.

Adapted from Sladyk, K. (2001). *OT exam review manual.* Thorofare, NJ: SLACK Incorporated and Sladyk, K. (2001). *OTA exam review manual.* Thorofare, NJ: SLACK Incorporated.

these feelings can seem overwhelming, but a few simple techniques might help. *Common Cognitive-Behavioral Techniques* (p. 163) suggests techniques to control anxiety while studying or during the exam itself. Review the chart for techniques that you can personalize. Remember that, just as you tell your clients, practice makes perfection. These cognitive-behavioral techniques must be consistently used to be effective.

Fieldwork or Life Issues Interfere with Studying

Some fieldwork sites are especially challenging, expecting students to perform all day and study for fieldwork all evening. These rich sites may be exhaust-

ing but likely very helpful in studying for the exam. While preparing for the next day of fieldwork, consider adding a few questions to your thinking about possible exam questions. When you find a handy chart or nice review in a book while investigating a fieldwork issue, mark the page with a note to return to when studying for the exam. Engage your supervisor in conversations about content questions you may have as demonstrated by the student Juan on p. 160.

Sometimes other life issues, such as crises, interfere with fieldwork and studying for the exam. Contact your AFWC as soon as possible so an individualized action plan can be put in place. Request the assistance of family and friends who might be able to help. Use student services back on campus, such as the aca-

COUNTDOWN CALENDAR

Month: _____

Sunday	Monday	Tuesday	Wednesday	Thursday	Friday	Saturday

COMMON COGNITIVE-BEHAVIORAL TECHNIQUES

Yell, "Stop!": Either out loud or to yourself. This technique stops the repeating thoughts of failure. Each time the thought returns, yell stop again.

Visualize success: Picture yourself taking the exam at the testing center with confidence and peace.

Take a 5-minute mind trip: Imagine yourself doing something pleasurable: sitting on a beach, walking in warm rain, or enjoying a beautiful vista. After a few minutes, remind yourself that it is okay to leave this place and return to studying because you can always come back later.

Set up a stress-free study place: Reduce distractions; study in a place you do not sleep or entertain. Adjust the light to your specific level. Buy and wear earplugs from a local hardware store. Take the earplugs with you on testing day.

Relaxation exercises: You likely learned how to teach your OT consumers how to relax, now practice it yourself. Take deep cleansing breaths, in through your nose, out through your mouth. Tense and relax muscle groups beginning with your toes and working your way up to your face.

Self-talk: Talk to yourself in a positive manner. After trying a relaxation exercise, remind yourself how relaxed you feel and how great you are doing.

Physically move: Sometimes just walking or dancing around can relieve the physical symptoms of anxiety. Find a song that is motivating and blast it out loud while dancing up a storm.

demic center, counseling services, or other programs. Remember that most crises pass with time, and you just need a plan to help that time pass.

Summary

This chapter presented practical suggestions to formulate a study plan to prepare during fieldwork for the NBCOT exam. Because studying is not new to the college experience, techniques that prepare students for the integrative nature of the certification exam were the focused study methods. Because the certification exam carries financial and personal pressures, it is important that students develop an individualized study plan early in level II fieldwork.

References

American Occupational Therapy Association. (1994). Uniform terminology for occupational therapy. *Am J Occup Ther, 48*(11), 1047-1059.

American Occupational Therapy Association. (2001). *Occupational therapy practice framework (draft)*. Bethesda, MD: Author.

Cottrell, R. (2001). National occupational therapy certification exam. Available as part of International Educational Resources' exam review workshop.

Dundon, H. D. (1988). *Examination review: Occupational therapy*. East Norwalk, CT: Appleton & Lange.

Ellis, D. (2000). *Becoming a master student*. Boston, MA: Houghton Mifflin Company.

Johnson, C., Lurch, A., & DeAngelis, T. (2001). *The occupational therapy examination review guide* (2nd ed.). Philadelphia, PA: F. A. Davis.

Moyers, P. (1999). *The guide to occupational therapy practice*. Bethesda, MD: American Occupational Therapy Association.

National Board for Certification in Occupational Therapy. (1999). *Study guide for the OT[A] certification examination*. Gaithersburg, MD: Author.

Reed, K. (2000). *Quick reference to occupational therapy*. Gaithersburg, MD: Aspen Publications.

Sladyk, K. (1999). *OT study cards in a box*. Thorofare, NJ: SLACK Incorporated.

Sladyk, K. (2001). *OTA exam review manual*. Thorofare: NJ: SLACK Incorporated.

Sladyk, K., & Sheckley, B. (2000). Clinical reasoning and reflective practice. *Occupational Therapy in Health Care, 13*(1), 11-22.

Chapter 15

Developing Your Professional Portfolio

JoAnne Wright, PhD, OTR

Developing a professional portfolio provides a constructive way to organize and document professional endeavors throughout your career (Alsop, 1995b). An excellent time to start your portfolio is as a student, either during the academic portion or during fieldwork. It is a way to present yourself to a future employer in a professional manner. If a portfolio is started early on in your career, it will eventually have the added benefit of reminding you just how much you really do know and how much you have progressed as an occupational therapy practitioner. By the end of this chapter, you will understand the following:

⟹ The different types of professional portfolios and their uses.

⟹ The benefits of using a portfolio in planning and evaluating the progress of professional goals and building self-esteem.

⟹ How to use a portfolio in presenting yourself to others including, but not limited to, prospective employers, supervisors, and promotion committees.

⟹ The importance of a resource portfolio as an aid to treatment planning.

WHAT IS A PORTFOLIO?

In general, a portfolio is a collection of materials or information. You have probably heard of someone's stock portfolio, which is a collection of investments, stocks, and bonds. An artist's portfolio is a very practical way in which to show his or her talent through a collection of examples. Sometimes, it is the actual work, and sometimes it is copies of the work.

Professional portfolios are now used in many disciplines including teaching, nursing, business, and occupational therapy (Alsop, 1995a, 1995b; Crist, Wilcox, & McCarron, 1998; Deitz, 1995; Marsh & Lasky, 1984). There are several different types of portfolios, and this chapter details a system that is tailored for an OT or OTA student who is transitioning into his or her professional role or who has just made the transition. In addition, the National Board for Certification in Occupational Therapy (NBCOT) is developing a portfolio program to document practitioners continuing competency. This new program is expected to begin with 2002 NBCOT renewals. It is never too late to start organizing—using the concepts of a portfolio—but the sooner you begin, the more beneficial it can be, and the easier it will be to get started (Bossers, Kernaghan, Merla, & Van Kessel, 1999).

The model presented in this chapter with the components of a presentation portfolio and a resource portfolio provide flexibility and a way to organize information about yourself and the information you will use as a therapist.

The first type, or the *presentation portfolio*, has two components. The first component is a collection of work you have produced during your academic coursework and your level II experiences, as well as reflections (Alsop, 1995b; Bossers et al., 1999; Crist, 1997; Deitz, 1995). It is a collection of information that is about you as a professional.

The second component of the presentation portfolio is a condensed version of your collection of materials, giving you a presentable compilation of your professional accomplishments. Your résumé will get you in the door for an interview and give your prospective employers a quick overview of who you are and what you have done. A well-done presentation portfolio will help them decide that based on the creative things you have done and the experiences you have had, you are unique from the other applicants and should be strongly considered.

The second type, or *resource portfolio*, is a way to organize the information you have collected in school and during your level II fieldwork experiences. Both the presentation and resource portfolio types will be discussed in greater detail.

The Presentation Portfolio: Component One

The first component of this portfolio should be thought of as the gathering place for materials related to your endeavors as a professional—although, as a student, you have been doing professional things all along during the education process. Your method of filing this information needs to make sense to you. You will most likely keep some of the information, such as your résumé, on your computer. It is a good idea to have a hard copy in your files just in case your computer crashes. There is no set list of what to gather, and if you sit down, you can probably make a list of what you think is important pretty easily. Others have recommended collecting some of the following while in school (Bossers et al., 1999; Crist et al., 1998):

➡ Copies of transcripts.

➡ Awards and certificates of completion.

➡ Well-done, graded assignments.

➡ Projects you have done.

➡ Presentations.

➡ Extracurricular activities.

➡ Courses other than regular ones.

While on your fieldwork, you will have opportunities for which you will want to add documentation to your portfolio. These might include the following:

➡ Fieldwork evaluation form.

➡ Long-term and short-term professional goals.

➡ Projects.

➡ Presentation.

➡ Special recognition.

➡ List of types of clients with whom you have worked.

➡ Unsolicited letters from clients, supervisors, etc.

➡ Copies of certifications (CPR, continuing education).

In documenting your professional activities, some might be represented better with pictures or videos.

Keep in mind that it is better to keep too much than to throw something out that may be of value later.

As you collect and organize these items, it is important to reflect on how these relate to your professional goals and what the event or project has meant to you as an occupational therapy practitioner. Bossers et al. (1999) consider it one of the most important parts of putting a portfolio together. As you reflect, it is helpful to make notes of how this has helped you grow as a professional and/or the most significant things you have learned. This will help preserve the richness of the experience for later when you are looking through your portfolio.

Reflection is probably even more important as you put together pieces of your complete portfolio into what this chapter describes as the second component of the presentation portfolio.

The Presentation Portfolio: Component Two

It would be silly to load your file folders filled with the items gathered for your presentation portfolio into a suitcase and head for a job interview. That is where the second component of the presentation portfolio comes into play. This is where you pull together the best, most representative sample of who you are and what you have done as a professional up to this point. You may believe that as a fieldwork student, there is nothing to put there, but, if you have been collecting, as described in component one, you will be surprised by what you have accomplished. This also will feed into your confidence as a beginning practitioner or show you what you need to start doing, if you have not already done so to this point.

Items that you would bring together might include but certainly are not limited to the following:

- Résumé (see Chapter 16).
- Page with long-term and short-term professional goals.
- List of clients with whom you have worked (mark those with whom you did something very creative and show it later in the portfolio).
- Projects.
- Presentations.
- Samples of your written work, etc.

Think of this as similar to showing pictures from your latest travel adventure to friends (face it, therapy school is an adventure). You have 40 rolls of 36-picture film (40 x 36 = 1440). You like each one, and each has a very particular meaning because you were there. Your friends most likely would enjoy seeing 50 of the best pictures, and after that, their tolerance and interest would drop off dramatically. Your job is to find those 50 best pictures for your friends. Likewise, in setting up your presentation portfolio, your job is to find those "few best" examples of what you have done and who you are as a professional.

The portfolio should be informative and interesting. Try to keep it professional looking, and avoid making it cutesy. This is a professional portfolio and not an example of scrapbooking. There is a fine line between

keeping it interesting and making it a craft project. You can reduce your portfolio while still providing a maximum amount of information by making lists for some of your accomplishments. An example would be to list the presentations and in-services you have given at the beginning of that particular section of the presentation portfolio. Then, in that same section, go into more detail regarding the best presentation, either through pictures (if available and appropriate), outlines, and/or handouts.

As you add each item, use this time to carefully reflect on what you have gained from the experience and what you have contributed. You may be asked more specific questions during your interview, and you will be prepared to answer. It also provides the additional bonus of helping you to realize just how much you have learned and done. It is a great self-esteem builder. As you continue as a practitioner, it will also help you to take stock of what you have done and if you are developing yourself according to your long- and short-term goals. Crist et al. (1998) also suggest that you keep your portfolios as an historical record to look back on as the years progress. Again, this is a good tool to encourage reflection.

Although the organizational style and the presentation of the professional portfolio are up to you, if you have questions, it is a good idea to talk to your mentors and get their ideas. They are a bit further down the professional development road and may have additional suggestions.

One of the most important rules to remember as you put your presentation portfolio together is do not lie, inflate, or exaggerate the information. You may be asked to elaborate, and if you then minimize it or describe it as it really happened, you will have compromised your credibility to the person doing the interview. Just as important, you need to honestly describe what you have done and not minimize your part in an event or your creativity.

One of the best ways to put your portfolio together is to use a thin three-ring binder. It is up to you if you want to use page protectors. The goal is to make it easy to look through and to quickly get a sense of what you have to offer. Both components of the presentation portfolio are important in accomplishing this goal.

The Resource Portfolio

You are probably now in possession of either several notebooks, one for each class you have completed in school, or file folders, or a combination. There are probably a number of loose papers. This compilation may range from being very organized with indexes and cross-referencing to being a couple of stacks in the corner of your room that topple frequently or some type of filing system in between these two examples. Much of the information is very valuable as you begin to practice as a therapist, and it can be used in a variety of situations. At this point, as you begin your career, it would be beneficial to go through that stack and organize it for practice rather than by each class.

There are a couple of reasons why it is beneficial to sort through all this information now. If you are still on fieldwork and have yet to take the certification exam, it is a way to informally review what knowledge you have gained and also start figuring out what you need to restudy in depth for the exam. Another reason is that no matter how organized your files are from school, you are entering a time where the information may require a more comprehensive way of filing or cross-referencing so that it is easier to find resources quickly when you are working. The key to organizing this information is to use a system that makes sense to you and is relatively simple. If it does not really follow how you think or is too cumbersome, it is likely you will not keep your portfolio up, and it will not really be much use to you.

This chapter will give suggestions and possibilities, but the ultimate organizational structure will be what works best for you. You may also find that you change that system a few years down the line. I started with my resources in large binders by subject with tabs and a cross-referencing index. After being a therapist for a few years, I decided that I wanted to use file folders and a filing cabinet. Neither one is right or wrong; my organizational style changed, as did the square footage of my living arrangement and the amount of material stored.

How to Get Started

No matter what system you decide to use, getting started is pretty much the same.

- ➡ Decide what type of organization you will use.
- ➡ Obtain the necessary materials.
- ➡ File the materials.
- ➡ List topics and where they are.
- ➡ Continue to update the files.

Decide What Type of Organization to Use

As has been suggested before, there are several ways to organize your materials. You will want to decide how to file the information; it might be by type of treatment or age group or by type of assessment. Use whatever makes sense to you, but take the time to really think through whether everything can be filed and retrieved with the system you choose. If you do not know what will work best, use the mentor model, and ask one or more therapists with whom you have worked and respect.

Obtain the Necessary Materials

Having decided your organizational framework, the next step is to gather the materials. File folders or binders work well. There are several types of files ranging from the colorful milk crate types to metal or wooden file cabinets. Try to choose something that has the capacity to expand to hold at least 20% more information than what you currently have to file.

File the Materials

With your organizational plan in place, you are now ready to start filing. Go through your materials and discard any notes or items that no longer make sense to you. File the other items, and, as you do so, make a list of the items that may have an application in a different category.

List Topics and Where They Are

You may want to use index cards or separate sheets of paper to note the item that has a couple of applications. Place the reference in the sections that do not have the actual item so you are able find it where it is located. You can then cross-reference the information in a number of places so you can find it easily. Besides the hard copy file, you may want to set up an indexing system using a computer program. This may be as simple as a list, or you may want to use a program that you can cross-reference with and be able to find the information by keyword. It is your call. Some find it useful, while others are better off with just the hard files.

Continue to Update the Files

As you read articles from professional journals, attend continuing education programs or workshops, and develop your own forms and evaluations, keep adding these to your files. Your occupational therapy career will probably lead you into treatment arenas you had no idea you might be in, and you just never know what might come in handy. To keep your resource file useful, you will want to update it at least yearly. Often, you come across useful items that you have forgotten you had in your file, and it gives you a chance to discard dated information.

SUMMARY

This chapter has shown how the presentation portfolio can be used to show yourself and others what has been accomplished regarding professional growth in skills and opportunities. The resource portfolio is another way to organize professional materials to be ready at hand as new treatment situations arise. Both are ways to remind the occupational therapy practitioner of how much he or she has grown professionally, whether the time frame is at the end of his or her occupational therapy education or a few years out.

REFERENCES

Alsop, A. (1995a). The professional portfolio—purpose, process and practice, Part 2: Producing a portfolio from experiential learning. *British Journal of Occupational Therapy, 58*(8), 337-340.

Alsop, A. (1995b). The professional portfolio—purpose, process and practice, Part 1: Portfolios and professional practice. *British Journal of Occupational Therapy, 58*(7), 299-302.

Bossers, A., Kernaghan, J., Merla, L., & Van Kessel, M. (1999). Portfolios: A powerful professional development tool. *OT Now, July/August,* 11-13.

Crist, P. (1997). Portfolios: A new aid to employment. *Advance for Occupational Therapists, 13*(19), 4.

Crist, P., Wilcox, B., & McCarron, K. (1998). Transitional portfolios: Orchestrating our professional competence. *Am J Occup Ther, 52*(9), 729-736.

Deitz, M. (1995). Using portfolios as a framework for professional development. *Journal of Staff Development, 16*(2), 40-43.

Marsh, H., & Lasky, P. (1984). The professional portfolio: Documentation of prior learning. *Nurs Outlook, 32*(5), 264-267.

Chapter 16

WRITING A RÉSUMÉ AND INTERVIEWING

Georganna Joary Miller, MEd, OTR

Let's face it, everything you have been doing up to this point has been working toward reaching your personal goal, which is getting a job as an occupational therapy practitioner. Much time and effort has been spent learning how to develop intervention plans for clients in order to help them achieve a goal of occupational independence or satisfaction. Now, you should begin to put time and effort into developing an intervention plan for yourself to help you reach your goal of occupational satisfaction. It is time to design a game plan for obtaining that first job as a real OT or OTA. Your academic program and fieldwork sites are designed to prepare you for the roles you will undertake as an occupational therapy practitioner. An equally important preparation must be undertaken to prepare you for the task of searching for and successfully obtaining gainful employment. Employment goal setting and developing the needed skills to reach that goal of becoming employed as an occupational therapy practitioner are the focus of this chapter.

By the end of this chapter, you will know the following:

➠ How to develop a résumé.

➠ When to send the résumé.

➠ How to find places to send the résumé.

➠ How to prepare for an interview.

➠ What should occur during the interview.

Writing the Résumé

Finding the right employment match for you and the employer is not a simple process and often is not given the time and consideration by all those involved in making this important decision. Taking a job for the primary goal of securing a paycheck can be an expensive mistake for both you and an employer. The emotional cost that you might incur if the employment situation does not work out well can be devastating. Depression from job dissatisfaction and stress from job pace, job insecurity, and job demands not only affect one's psyche but also impact one's physical well-being. Being prone to catching colds, influenza, and headaches is often a first indication that stress from the work environment is attacking your immune system. Job-hunting is also expensive if you have to take unpaid time off from a bad job situation to look for a better one.

The mistake can prove costly to a desperate employer who hires the first warm body to walk in the door just to solve a critical staffing shortage. This may result in additional workloads for the entire department. All staff may share the responsibility of dealing with the mess created by hiring an employee who may not be well trained or well suited to the needs of the facility. Staff turnover is a financially and emotionally draining expense for an occupational therapy department. The costs of advertising, staff and management time needed for interviewing, hiring, training new personnel, possible use of expensive agency therapists to cover caseloads, as well as paying current staff overtime to cover for the shortage of personnel can wreak havoc on a department's fiscal budget.

Until the 1980s, occupational therapy managers may have received only one or two unsolicited resumes per month across their desks. If the facility advertised an open position, the occupational therapy manager might have received only three resumes in response to the ad. Times have changed, though, and during the 1990s, an increase in the number of occupational therapy educational programs produced an expanded supply of OT and OTA graduates. This was complicated further with changes in reimbursement and the resulting downsizing of many occupational therapy departments. Consequently, the numbers of occupational therapy job openings declined significantly by the late 1990s. Occupational therapy managers suddenly were faced with the new dilemma of a steady stream of resumes arriving in the mail and numerous qualified applicants from whom to select for any one opening. Though the job market is improving after a severe slump in 1998 and 1999, a competitive environment remains as occupational therapy practitioners look for jobs, especially positions with well-respected facilities or agencies. This competitive environment can be a friendlier battleground if it is met with a well-prepared résumé. Providing prospective employers with a quality résumé that catches the attention of the reader and presents a clear and positive picture of you is the challenge at hand.

The traditional viewpoint of the résumé's function is to serve as a record, for initial contact or statement and an inclusion-elimination device. Its main purpose is to obtain an interview, not a job (Drafke, 1994). This is a key message to remember and should serve as the inspiration for you to take care and consideration when developing your résumé. Following the guidelines in this chapter should prevent your résumé from being tossed aside or overlooked.

Fox (2001) presents a rather stark, but accurate, concept about resumes. He labels you as a marketable product and your résumé as your sales literature. He goes on to assert the two purposes of a résumé: "1) to be intriguing enough to get you an interview; and 2) to reaffirm in a tailored way, after your interview, how hiring you solves the hirer's problem" (p. 11). So, the résumé needs to catch the employer's attention and convince him or her that you are the answer to his or her prayers.

Throughout occupational therapy school, you probably heard more than one professor respond with the phrase, "there is no one right way of doing this" when discussing aspects of the occupational therapy process, such as evaluation or intervention. This phrase is often frustrating for students to hear because, especially earlier in their careers, they are often searching for the best answer. This mantra, however, is a theme that is also repeated when discussing the format for a résumé. There is no one right way of organizing a résumé. If five managers are asked to review one résumé, five ideas on how to format a résumé will likely be offered. The format of a résumé, however, is probably not as critical as the content. Furthermore, the same five managers can debate the issue of content. Having said that, there are a few general guidelines for format and content that can be followed when creating a résumé.

First of all, there are generally considered two basic types of resumes: chronological and functional (Drafke, 1994). Newly graduated, entry-level occupational therapy practitioners will do well to use the chronological résumé format. A functional résumé is considered better suited for experienced individuals with work experiences that are closely matched to the positions for which they are applying. When writing a chronological résumé, it is important to keep the length short to ensure that it is read in its entirety by managers whose schedules do not allow the luxury of in-depth reading. Examples of chronological resumes are provided to help you consider a method of formatting your information (see *Sample Resumes A and B* on pp. 176-178). These resumes have similar content headings and distinct sections for education, work experience, and professional activities. Each should be examined carefully to note that the information varies in illustrating the individual's unique life experiences that are of interest to a potential employer.

Fox (2001) suggests writing an individual résumé for each target facility. This is especially important when the facility to which you are sending the résumé has a specialized population or service area. When tailoring a résumé for a unique audience, expand the details of information relevant to that setting and omit some of the general information in order to keep the length of the résumé to two pages. For example, elaborate on your fieldwork experiences to show that the skills you developed there would be readily transferred to an employment setting. Now, carefully describe those experiences and responsibilities for the reader to improve your chances of obtaining an interview. Another instance that might call for a tailor-made résumé is when additional educational experiences have been obtained. Directly relate any specialty certifications, continuing education, or additional degrees in another area, such as education or psychology, to the advertised job description.

As a new graduate, you may be looking for a general, entry-level position where specific skills are not sought in the job description and are not an important selling point to the employer. Instead, an employer may be more interested in an employee who is willing to learn and accept facility-specific training. Jackson and Jackson (1996) encourage new grads to find a way to demonstrate willingness and a passion for learning, as well as a commitment to working hard when faced with various work situations. How to show this on paper is the real challenge. Perhaps the area of investigation and quality of your research paper is an accurate reflection of your ability to see a difficult task to completion. Maybe the various responsibilities you accepted in a summer job show your willingness to take risks and assume authority. Briefly identifying specific work tasks involved in a prior job may give an employer the impression you are not afraid to venture into new horizons.

When you were applying for acceptance to an occupational therapy educational program, you may have created a résumé or autobiography to highlight your assets. To show the occupational therapy program selection committee that you were a well-rounded individual with varied interests, skills, and leadership experiences, you probably listed your involvement in extra-curricular activities during high school. Creating a similar image for an occupational therapy employer can be achieved by listing the activities in which you were involved during occupational therapy school. Such involvement will indicate the ability to lead a balanced life.

Drafke (1994) identifies five primary character traits that should be included in a résumé: a desire to work, a work ethic, flexibility (in working times), ambition, and dedication. All five of these traits can often be illustrated concurrently on a résumé. For example, not only does the fact that you may have worked a part-time job while in occupational therapy school demonstrate a desire to work, but a potential employer could also form an opinion about your work ethic from your continued volunteer work and active membership in school clubs and professional organizations. When looking at your résumé, an employer might decide you are flexible by looking at the different shifts you worked in a summer job or that you were able to work on a variety of units or assigned areas.

Drafke (1994) suggests ambition can be demonstrated by identifying previous work experience, promotions, advancement in professional organizations, and advancement in community or volunteer organizations. Being involved in a variety of clubs or organizations, and especially holding any leadership positions, such as secretary, president, or committee chair, can tell a prospective employer that you are ambitious and that you are able to use time management skills to balance numerous responsibilities.

Clubs can also illustrate your dedication and respect for a balance in life interests, especially if the clubs or organizations listed on your résumé are related to interests not only in occupational therapy but outside the profession as well. Dedication to the profession of occupational therapy usually can be documented by listing memberships in the American Occupational Therapy Association (AOTA), any state and local occupational therapy associations, related special interest sections, and groups for selected diagnoses, populations, intervention approaches, etc. (e.g., National Association for Therapeutic Horseback Riding, National Association for Aquatic Therapy, or National Association for Mental Illness).

In the two sample resumes provided (see *Sample Resumes A and B*), the students list both level I and level II fieldworks with details of selected experiences or activities they were involved in during their experiences. Doing this can show a potential employer what diagnoses and intervention techniques you have observed and participated in that may be further

SAMPLE RÉSUMÉ A

KATE WASA-STUDENT
3823 Academic Drive, Cincinnati, OH 45207   (513) 555-3824

EDUCATION/HONORS
Xavier University, Cincinnati, Ohio
B.S. in Occupational Therapy
December 2001
- Presidential Scholarship Award for academics, 1997-2001
- Dean's List, 1997-2001
- Alpha Sigma Nu, 1999 inductee
- Jesuit honor society for academics, leadership, and service
- Mortar Board, 2000 inductee
- National honor society for academics and leadership
Research participation, 2000-2001: "The Primary Needs of Greater Cincinnati's Homeless Population in Relation to Occupational Therapy"
- Presented at National Conference of Undergraduate Research, Lexington, KY, 2001
- Presented at Xavier University 2001 Celebration of Student Research, Cincinnati, OH
- Presented at Xavier University Occupational Therapy Research Symposium, 2001

WORK EXPERIENCE
Level II fieldwork
- Community Occupational Therapy Services, Memphis, TN; psychosocial setting June 25- September 14, 2001
- Greenville Hospital System, Greenville, SC; physical disabilities setting September 25- December 14, 2001

Level I fieldwork
- Mercy Fairfield Hospital, Fall 2000, Cincinnati, OH
  Acute care physical disabilities setting. Observed Neonatal Intensive Care practice with craniosacral therapy. Worked with CVA, TKR, THR, autism, cancer, premature infants.
- Habilitation Services, Spring 2000, Cincinnati, OH
  Pediatric setting. Used Willbarger techniques and Sensory Integration frame of reference treatments
- William Mitchell Center, Fall 1999, Cincinnati, OH
  Psychosocial setting. Ran groups for adult day program. Worked with individuals with schizophrenia, depression, bipolar, MR/DD diagnoses.

OTHER WORK EXPERIENCE
Russell's Tuxedos, Cincinnati, OH
- Assistant Manager, May 1998- August 1998
- Sales Associate, March 1995- June 1999
Xavier University Summer Service Internship, Cincinnati, OH May 2000- August 2000
- Summer Service Intern
- Project Connect Educational Services
- Summer Camp Intern, Provided educational services to children who were living in homeless shelters and who attended a summer camp through Project Connect. Chaperoned various excursions.
NORCEN Behavioral Health Systems, Cincinnati, OH May 1999- August 1999
- Activities Assistant, Ran groups and activities for adult day program

PROFESSIONAL MEMBERSHIPS
American Occupational Therapy Association, August 1998-present.
- Attended national conference 1999 and 2001.
Xavier University Student Occupational Therapy Association, Fall 1998-May 2001
- Treasurer, Fall 2000-May 2001
- Co-coordinator of the Drop Inn Center Shelter outreach program

SAMPLE RÉSUMÉ A (CONTINUED)

Ohio Occupational Therapy Association, August 1999-2000
  • Attended and assisted on hospitality committee at state conference, Sept. 1999
SPECIAL SKILLS
Computer: WordPerfect, Microsoft Word, Microsoft Excel, and Microsoft Power Point
Assistive Technology: Fabrication of equipment and use of computer programming, head pointer, Intellikeys, wheelchair adaptations, head mouse
CPR certified
10-week course on Hand Therapy
10-week course on Holistic Health Integration
10-week course on Driver Evaluation and Training
ACTIVITIES
Xavier University Campus Ministry, September 1997-May 2001
  • Retreat leader
  • Small group leader
Muskie's Own Recruitment Effort, Xavier University, Fall 1997-May 2001
  • Tour guide
Board of Ambassadors, Xavier University, January 1999- May 2001
College Friends, Xavier University, Fall 1997- May 2001
  • Mentor to local elementary students
  • Vice President, Fall 1999-May 2001
St. Vincent de Paul, Cincinnati, OH, Fall 1999- May 2000
Tutor at St. Mark's Elementary, Cincinnati, OH for kindergarten age children. Mentor for 6-year-old over the summer break, May-September 1999

SAMPLE RÉSUMÉ B

Bryan B. Hunting

Local Address (Until 4/20/02)   **Permanent Address:**
1393 Waverly Ave. #2   3451 Robinwood Ln.
Norwood, OH 45515   Millersburg, OH 55421
(505) 555-7243   (505) 555-5145
OBJECTiVE   Seeking an entry-level position in occupational therapy.
EDUCATION Cincinnati State Technical and Community College, Cincinnati, Ohio
            Associate Degree in Occupational Therapy Assisting
            Graduation, April 2001
            Summa Cum Laude
            Dean's List 8/8 Quarters
CLINICAL EXPERIENCE
Fieldwork Level II
Wadsworth Rittman Hospital, Wadsworth, OH; June-September 2001
Riley Hospital, Indianapolis, IN; September-December 2001

Fieldwork Level I
Eastgate Healthcare Center, Cincinnati, OH; Fall 1999 (Geriatrics)
Cincinnati Occupational Therapy Institute (COTI), Cincinnati, OH; Spring 1999 (Pediatrics)
Northern Kentucky Rehabilitation HEALTHSOUTH, Edgewood, KY Fall 2000 (Adult Rehab)

SAMPLE RÉSUMÉ B (CONTINUED)

RELATED WORK EXPERIENCE

One-on-one Aide with Autistic Child, Cincinnati, OH; June 2000-May 2001
- Planned and facilitated activities to help achieve occupational therapy, speech therapy, and educational goals
- Collaborated with and assisted occupational therapist, speech therapist, aquatic instructor, and classroom aide

Habilitation Assistant, Society for Handicapped Citizens, Wadsworth, OH; Summer 1999
- Assisted adults with mental retardation in carrying out daily living activities
- Implemented and documented daily and weekly programs supporting individualized habilitation programs (IHPs)

Server, Cracker Barrel, Akron, OH; Summer 1997, Summer 1998

PROFESSIONAL INVOLVEMENT

American Occupational Therapy Association (AOTA) member; 1998-present
CSTCC Student Occupational Therapy Association member; 1998-2001
AOTA National Conference, attendee, Indianapolis, IN; 1999, Philadelphia, PA; 2001
Ohio Occupational Therapy Association (OOTA) Conference, attendee, Cincinnati, OH; 1999

ACTIVITIES

HOSTS (Helping One Student to Succeed), Volunteer, Burton Elementary, Cincinnati, OH; (2001)
Circle K, Community service connections club, Cincinnati, OH, Member 1997-present; VP 1999-2001; Service chair 1998-1999
Navigators Ministry, Cincinnati, OH, Member 1997-2001; Bible study leader 1998-1999; Worship leader 1999-2000
COTI Volunteer, Cincinnati, OH; OT/Speech Therapy summer camp; summer 2000
Faith and Service Theme House member (1999-2000)
CSTCC Occupational Therapy Program Student Advisory Board Member; 1999-2001
Volunteer, St. Francis Elementary, Reading is Xcellent, Cincinnati, OH; 1998-1999
CSTCC Soccer team 1999-2000, team captain 2000

HONORS

CSTCC Presidential Scholarship recipient, Cincinnati, OH 1999-2001
Ohio Community Colleges Honor Society Inducted 1999
Mortar Board (Inducted 2000)
Community Life Academic Award, recipient, CSTCC 1999-2000
Governor's Academic Excellence Recognition for Allied Health Student 2000
Christian Athlete's Award 2000

REFERENCES

Available upon request.

---

developed at your first job. An employer who is looking to future program development may be persuaded to hire you over another candidate simply based on the fact that you have an initial exposure to, albeit a limited understanding of, what a specific program essentially might entail. Sample Resumes A and B list "related work experiences" or "other work experiences." The various jobs listed in these sections show an employer that you may have work skills, such as dealing with the public, solving problems, following directions, or working independently. Involvement in such jobs may also point out specialized work skills that will complement an occupational therapy position. Any future employer will value previous experience in word processing and computers, operating selected equipment, public speaking, or leading groups.

Yet another area of interest to potential employers will be any research activity in which you engaged during occupational therapy school. Engaging in the research process is a highly valued skill, as it is widely thought to be essential to the survival and continued development of occupational therapy (Gilfoyle & Christiansen, 1987). Listing the title of any research projects in which you participated can give your résumé a "top of the pile" status, especially if the employer is intrigued by the topic or is interested in using similar ideas in his or her setting. Collaborative research efforts may further show evidence of your ability to work in a team or to be a team player. Having presented your research in any forum, such as at a local, state, or national conference, or as an in-service to a group of clinicians in order to meet a field-work requirement, has the potential to further impress a future employer. The various research presentations listed in *Sample Résumé A* under Education/Honors suggest the strong beginnings of a researcher engaged in scholarly work. A future employer may highly value such involvement in research dissemination for the validity it brings to the employer's institution, our clients, and our profession.

People often end the résumé with either a list of personal references or a line indicating that references are available upon request. Employers need to contact references for the purpose of verifying the accuracy of the information on the résumé and to have someone else validate that their decision to offer you a job is a good choice. Whichever method you choose to follow, you should personally contact the individuals before listing any names as references on your résumé and request their permission to list them as personal references. It is a good idea to let your references know specifically who might be calling them and what information you prefer that they do or do not share with the potential employer. Try to use references that can emphasize the variety of your personal qualities—for example, a professor who has taught you for more than one course and could attest to your ability to demonstrate initiative in independent learning and in working with other students on group assignments. Another reference should be a therapist who supervised you on fieldwork and can attest to your interaction skills with clients and professional disciplines. Last, a former employer should be listed as a reference, even if it is the night supervisor from McDonald's or a family you did babysitting for during the summer. These individuals could corroborate your willingness to accept and follow through on responsibilities, your dependability, and your flexibility in dealing with varying structure.

One last area of great debate in résumé writing rests in how many pages the résumé should be in length. Résumé gurus often defend the position of a single-page résumé (Drafke, 1994). Most managers will not complain that the résumé they received was two pages long, and certainly will not throw out a résumé simply because it did not meet the one-page rule. It may be easy for you to summarize your life highlights on just one page; however, if you are trying to portray an accurate picture of your ambition, dedication, and experience, one page may just not be enough paper. One note of advice, though, is to use a standard size 12 font. Do not try to decrease the font size just to make your content fit on one piece of paper. Does a size 10 font give a Freudian interpretation that you do not think very highly of yourself? On the other hand, do not go to the other extreme and have the font size appear as if you have a grandiose self-image. Finally, have several people read and proof your résumé for grammar and punctuation. Repeated proofreadings by several sources will further increase the accuracy. Typographical errors almost ensure your résumé will be placed at the bottom of the pile, or maybe even into a "circular file" status.

WRITING THE COVER LETTER

Fox (2001) argues that, in the business world, sending out resumes is passé and that it is better to make a telephone call to let an employer know who you are. In the *real world* of occupational therapy, it is still one of the best ways to attempt an initial contact with an occupational therapy employer. Making a "cold call" to an occupational therapy department in hopes of finding an occupational therapy manager who will take your phone call, listen to you introduce yourself, explain your career goals, and request an interview may actually do you more harm than good. Managers are often too busy to give you the attention you are hoping for and may be annoyed or impatient with your unanticipated interruption. Giving the occupational therapy manager the opportunity to open your cover letter and résumé, attend to it at his or her convenience, and return to it when he or she is looking for new staff may give you the inside advantage you are seeking.

So, go ahead and send a résumé, but not until you have written a worthy cover letter to preface the résumé you have spent hours perfecting. Be sure the cover letter is content specific and tailored to address the advertised need. Fox (2001) advises against addressing it "To Whom It May Concern" and adds that a cover letter with such a greeting could be considered junk mail. Find out the name of the individual who is in charge of hiring and interviewing for occupational therapy positions by calling the personnel department. This may take some persistence and patience to obtain information as you work your way through the phone maze of the facility or agency, but it is a good opportunity for you to profile your assertiveness skills. Explicitly state the position for which you are applying. The astute manager will easily detect a generic cover letter.

The cover letter should be one page in length and include the following basics:

➠ Date.

➠ Heading (the facility's name and address).

➠ Greeting (directly addressed to a real person, not "To Whom It May Concern" or "Dear Sir or Madam").

➠ Succinct body (mention your career objective; how you heard about the job; when you could interview; when you would be available to begin working; and direct the reader to your enclosed résumé).

➠ Signature (legibly written above a typed name that includes credentials).

Avoid mentioning any salary requests in your cover letter, as this is likely to come across more aggressive than assertive upon initial contact. This matter can be more appropriately addressed during the interview. Additionally, briefly include in the cover letter information such as previous work experience directly related to the position that might give you an edge over other applicants. In this way, you use the cover letter to draw attention to any specifics on the résumé that you do not want overlooked. End the cover letter with specific details of the best time and telephone number where you can be reached so that an interview can be arranged.

Finally, as with the résumé, typographical errors will generate an unfavorable impression to any future employer. Have someone else read and proof it several times for any errors in spelling and grammar. A cover letter cannot be proofed too many times.

A follow-up telephone call is recommended approximately 2 weeks after the cover letter and résumé was mailed to ensure it was received.

FINDING PLACES TO SEND YOUR RÉSUMÉ OR CALL FOR AN INTERVIEW

Once you have finished the final draft of your résumé, completed your cover letter, and made numer-

ous copies of each, you will want to circulate it to potential employers. There are numerous avenues you can pursue when making a decision about who should receive your résumé.

The Local Newspaper

Although this is frequently chosen as a place to start job-hunting, and is probably the easiest, it may not be the best option for finding the job of your dreams. Because not all employers advertise there, the newspaper definitely should not be the only option you use in your job search. In fact, many companies specifically avoid advertising in newspapers, thinking the realistic market is too limiting and not worthwhile. The opportunities listed below may take a little more energy, but are likely to be more productive toward achieving your goal of gainful employment. Use as many of these options as you can to improve your chances of securing a position more efficiently and in a timelier manner.

State and District Placement Chairs

Many state and local district-level occupational therapy associations have individuals who assume responsibility of being a "placement chair." This means that facilities that have job openings can call the placement chair and ask to have their vacant position posted for any occupational therapist who might be looking for employment. Using this service is usually offered free of charge to the facility and the therapist.

Journals

Looking in professional journals used to be one of the best ways to see the opportunities available in the job market, but the current cost constraints often prohibit advertising in journals for many occupational therapy departments. Across the country, many departments' fiscal budgets have been close-shaved as a result of the far-reaching changes in reimbursement. Another problem inherent with journal advertisements lies in the length of time that passes from when the employer submits the ad to the journal and when the journal is published and subsequently reaches your home. The advertised job may have been filled by the time you have the journal in your hand to read. When you use this avenue for job hunting, do not limit yourself by just reading the *American Journal of Occupational Therapy*. There may be job opportunities listed in other professional journals that are not necessarily identified as occupational therapy but that could be easily filled by an OT or OTA. In such case, you may just need to explain to the employer that your qualifications and education have prepared you for the job opening and the employer just needs to re-title the position to that of an occupational therapy practitioner to match your expertise. An example of this could be an ad for a rehabilitation generalist, an activity therapist, or a residence manager. The job description might involve the roles and responsibilities that are obviously in keeping with the training and education of an occupational therapy practitioner. Discuss with the employer how your educational preparation qualifies you for this position and that by hiring you and re-titling the job description, third-party reimbursement for your services might be a possible option for the facility to pursue.

Web Sites

Job-hunting on the Internet has become increasingly popular and can be an efficient resource to use. Again, do not limit yourself to just the familiar job-hunting sites such as jobhunter.com, monster.com, or headhunter.net. For example, log on to specific facilities' web sites and look for the connection to their personnel or human resources department. Here, you find a list of current job openings. Logging onto state occupational therapy association web sites may also give you a listing of job openings or placement chairs to contact. Also, check your state's Department of Labor, as they often have positions in state-run programs listed here first. Student members of AOTA can post their résumé on AOTA's website. This benefit puts your résumé in the premier occupational therapy web site.

Word of Mouth

Finding a job via word of mouth has been used for job-hunting since the beginning of time and continues to be a reliable means of obtaining leads on job openings. If you are looking for a job in an unfamiliar geographic area, you will need to be a little more creative to become part of "the loop." Becoming part of the loop suggests you are part of the professional network. One place to start networking with other occupational therapy practitioners is by attending district occupational therapy meetings, SIS section meetings, workshops, conferences, and in-services. Also, who you know can be important and helpful as a "friend of a friend of a friend" can provide you with inside information about who might be leaving a facility and creating a job opening in which you might be inter-

ested. Furthermore, an advantage to the word of mouth method is that often the speed with which you find out about possible job openings is a lot faster than the Internet or local newspapers. It is not uncommon for therapists to know that a colleague is leaving a position weeks before the employer is given the official resignation letter or clearance to post/advertise the opening.

College or University Career Services Centers

Colleges and universities often identify their career placement services as one of the unique benefits of attending their institution, although each university has its own unique name for this office. Helping graduates find jobs is frequently listed as an outcome objective for the institution. You invested a great deal of money to obtain a degree, so using the placement services they offer makes good sense and cents. Frequently, employers send announcements of job openings to the career services center or placement office, and you can access this information easily. The services are *usually* free of charge to the employer and the graduate. The career services center may also provide you with an opportunity to place your résumé on file with their office, so they can then provide it in response to future requests from potential employers.

Mailing to Occupational Therapy Departments or Facilities

Just because a facility has not listed a job in the newspaper, in a journal, or on the Internet does not mean it does *not* have a current opening or anticipate an opening in the near future. If you know of a facility or agency at which you would like to be employed, send your résumé to that site and follow up with a phone call. You may be surprised to coincidently find that the job opening was brought to the attention of the department supervisor the same day your résumé came in the mail.

Occupational therapy supervisors often keep resumes on file for several months after they have been received. Calls directed to occupational therapy department managers rather than to the human resources department may be more profitable. At times, individuals within the human resources departments may not have as much information about upcoming openings as the people directly involved in the day-to-day operations of an occupational therapy department.

Academic Fieldwork Coordinators

Who has more frequent contact with occupational therapy departments, facilities, agencies, and individual OTs and OTAs than an academic fieldwork coordinator (AFWC)? Often, when making the numerous calls to secure level I and level II fieldwork placements, the AFWC hears about job openings that are not yet publicized through the typical channels. The AFWCs are eager and happy to share this news with their graduates for two reasons. First, a fieldwork site that is fully staffed is more likely to take student interns, so the AFWC wants to keep job openings filled so a fieldwork placement can be maintained for future students. Second, most occupational therapy educational programs identify gainful employment status as one of their outcome objectives for their graduates. This is clearly a "win-win" situation for the AFWC, the graduate, the occupational therapy educational program, and the occupational therapy department, agency, or facility, so remember to use this important connection.

SELLING YOURSELF IN AN INTERVIEW

Earlier in this chapter, it was stated that the main purpose of the résumé was to obtain an interview, not necessarily a job. Well, now comes the step that is intended to get you a job—the interview. Interviewing for a job can be a humbling as well as an ego-boosting experience. Interviews give you a chance to identify your positive assets not only to a potential employer, but also to yourself. Each interview in which you participate has the potential for helping you gain further insight into your strengths and areas of concern. These insights can be a humbling experience. Interviews also can be ego-boosting in that they are enlightening and beneficial to your self-image no matter what the employment status outcome.

Questions You May Be Asked

The type and format of questions asked by an occupational therapy manager interviewing a potential therapist can vary considerably. The general content, however, tends to run along predictable themes. The following is a general list of sample questions that might be asked:

➠ How did you become interested in us?

➠ Why do you want to work here?

➠ What programs or services would you be able to start in our department?

➠ Tell me about a project you are proud of.

➠ What are you most proud of?

➠ What special interests/skills/goals do you have?

➠ Give an example of your resourcefulness.

➠ Give an example of your assertiveness or the most difficult situation you experienced at fieldwork, and how you handled it.

➠ Tell me something about yourself that I would not know from reading your résumé. *(Hint: make this something that would demonstrate good work skills, drive, or personal assets that are relevant to the position for which you are applying, such as that you have been financially responsible for your own education, but not personal items like how many pets you have or that you take care of four dogs and a horse.)*

Among a list of questions applicable to health care interviews, Adams (2001) includes the following:

➠ Which of your fieldwork experiences did you enjoy the most?

➠ What clients do you feel most comfortable working with?

➠ What clients do you feel least comfortable working with?

For the interview to result in a heightened state of self-awareness, you must prepare yourself fully for the journey. This begins with heeding a few simple words of wisdom regarding your personal appearance, body language, and interaction skills. Be sure to make a positive first impression by following these guidelines. First, when you meet the interviewer, offer a firm handshake and look the person in the eye while shaking hands (Dorio, 2000). Making eye contact is imperative in order to connect with the interviewer and to be perceived as self-confident.

The phrase "dress for success" should also receive your attention here. In his list of the most common interview complaints, Adams (2001) cited dressing too casual as a typical faux pas. So, when in doubt, error on the side of dressing up, although adhere to local norms and conservative guidelines when doing so. Sensible shoes, minimal jewelry, no visible tattoos or body piercing other than for one earring per ear, and well-groomed hair will be your safest bet. The rest of Adams' list (2001) of common interview complaints would be worth mentioning here as well: "The candidate

➠ did not research the company

➠ lacked enthusiasm

➠ did not ask questions

➠ was too fidgety

➡ did not make enough eye contact

➡ spoke too quickly

➡ spoke too much" (p.102)

Is it surprising to see that the complaint list is entirely focused on personal interaction skills? Use your personal interaction skills to make a good impression and to ensure the interview is successful. Although using strong interaction skills seems to be common sense, ignoring their impact or importance in an interview is inexcusable.

The employer and the potential employee should view interviews as a partnership venture. Equal responsibility must be shared by both parties to ensure that an accurate picture is painted of the job, the institution, and the candidate's ability. The employer has the responsibility of asking the standard routine battery of questions and describing the job position. The employer *should* show the candidate an actual job description and the essential job functions identified for the opening. The employer *should* offer the candidate the opportunity to look at the department's employee performance appraisal form. The performance appraisal form will give you an indication of what might be expected of you during the first year, such as productivity levels, additional department responsibilities, and margin for errors. The employer *should* offer the candidate a tour of the facility and a chance to observe other employees in action. The employer *should* offer the candidate an opportunity to interview and be interviewed by other staff in the department, especially staff who will be colleagues of the candidate. If the employer does not offer the above-mentioned opportunities to the candidate, then you, the candidate, *should* assume responsibility for obtaining them. Assertively request such information.

Your primary responsibility in the interview process is to come prepared to make the most of the valuable time being offered by the employer. Dorio (2000) emphasizes the need to show in the interview that you are someone who can do the job, will stick around, will fit in, and is likeable.

Jackson and Jackson (1996) report the most important qualities sought by someone who is hiring are resiliency/flexibility and leadership/initiative. How do you plan to show these qualities during your interview? Think of stories, illustrations, or examples to share in the interview that might demonstrate these qualities. You will find this time to be time well spent in preparing for an interview. Be sure to bring tangible items with you to the interview, such as a portfolio, copy of your research project, and examples of treatment plans or written work produced in school or during level II fieldwork. Preparation done prior to a job interview

can lessen your anxiety level before and during the interview, improving your image of being a mature and professional candidate. Take the time to complete the activities and checklists in *Preparing for the Interview* (p. 184) and *Interview Checklist* (p. 186) to improve your chances for success in the interview process.

Kief and Scheerer (2001) recommend that before you arrive in the occupational therapy department, you obtain information from the human resources or public relations office of the facility to answer the following questions. The items in parentheses will help you answer these questions more specifically.

➡ Who owns the facility? (and is it a nonprofit or a for-profit group?)

➡ Who is it affiliated with? (religious groups or a national health care system?)

➡ How many OTs and OTAs are working there?

➡ Number of beds or community caseload?

➡ Accreditations? (especially ones other than JCAHO)

➡ Population served?

➡ Research support? (or demands?)

➡ Get a copy of the Mission Statement and Philosophy of the institution.

You need to understand that there are certain questions you do not have to answer. Laws prohibit potential employers from asking confidential, personal information prior to employment. Not all interviewers are familiar with the laws and/or fail to follow the law. This is often done unknowingly and without intentional malice. In such a case, you need to be aware of questions that are and are not lawful. Drafke (1994) cites various authors and sources to outline questions that cannot be asked in the interview, such as the following:

➡ Marital status.

➡ Family plans.

➡ Sexual orientation.

➡ Age.

➡ Ethnic background.

➡ Race.

➡ Religion.

➡ Disability.

If you encounter questions directed toward any of the above issues, you may redirect the line of questioning. This may be awkward for you and the interviewer. Dorio (2000) suggests methods for dealing with such inappropriate questions. For example, if the interviewer asks if you are married, you might reply

PREPARING FOR THE INTERVIEW

The following questions are presented to generate potential content areas that will allow a future employer to see your strengths and get to know your attitudes, skills, and beliefs.

Who are you?

List three projects you worked on either independently or with a group that you are proud of having produced.

Example of a possible answer: "I co-led a cooking group for five clients with MR/DD in my level I fieldwork experience. I was able to plan the activity for four different sessions, took responsibility for obtaining all the supplies, and documented the clients' performance after each session. It was fun for the clients and for me, and the entire staff including the unit managers complimented me on how well it went."

1.

2.

3.

List three personal characteristics (strengths) about yourself that would be an asset to any OT department or potential employer.

Example of a possible answer: "I am a very detail-oriented person. I like to organize workspace for efficiency and take pride in having my environment look neat and orderly."

1.

2.

3.

List three personal characteristics (weaknesses) that are currently in a rebuilding phase, and identify what action plans you have established to resolve these issues.

Example of a possible answer: "I have trouble being assertive sometimes. I am trying to change this by reading books on assertiveness techniques and making a goal of practicing assertiveness at least three times a week with my friends and peers."

1.

2.

3.

PREPARING FOR THE INTERVIEW (CONTINUED)

List three technical skills that you bring to this position that would be an asset to the department.

Example: "I am computer literate in word processing (Microsoft Word), data analysis (Excel) software, assistive technology hardware for computer input (Intellikeys and Co:Writer), and presentation software (PowerPoint).

1.

2.

3.

Who do you want to be?

Identify three areas of specialization (e.g., populations, diagnoses, frames of reference, intervention methods) that intrigue or interest you, and state an action plan that you might pursue to develop your skill or knowledge base for each.

Example: "I want to learn more about hippotherapy. I am going to search the web for local organizations and contact one for information and possibly begin volunteering there."

1.

2.

3.

Identify any future career goals by answering each of these questions respectively:

Example: "In 1 year, I see myself supervising level I fieldwork students. In 3 years, I see myself being a fieldwork coordinator. In 5 years, I see myself being NDT certified. In 10 years, I see myself working in a private practice group."

Where do you see yourself in 1 year?

Where do you see yourself in 3 years?

Where do you see yourself in 5 years?

Where do you see yourself in 10 years?

(Note: Be honest with these answers. Do not just give lip service to what you think the potential employer wants to hear. If you do not see yourself as a staff therapist working in the same setting in 5 years, but rather see yourself working in a different system, say so. Employers realize that many therapists need to try other work areas in order to stay energized or motivated.)

INTERVIEW CHECKLIST

Before you leave for the interview, ask yourself these questions:
➡ Do I have extra copies of my résumé with me (in case the manager cannot find the résumé you sent or to hand to additional people who interview you at the facility)?
➡ Do I have my list of questions to ask the employer?
➡ Do I have my list of strengths, weaknesses, and goals with me?
➡ Do I look like a professional (appropriately dressed)?
➡ Do I have a map/address of where I am going?
➡ Do I have correct change to make a telephone call, the phone number, and name of who I am to meet, just in case I get lost or delayed?

Before ending the interview, ask yourself these questions:
➡ Have I seen a job description and essential job functions? In other words, do I have a clear idea of what this job entails?
➡ Have I seen the performance appraisal form? In other words, what will be expected of me the first year in order to keep this job and get a pay raise?
➡ Have I received a tour of the facility? In other words, do I have a clear picture of what my physical work environment will look like?
➡ Have I talked to the staff or made arrangements to do this at a later date? In other words, do I know who the people are who will be my coworkers/peers, and do I have an initial idea as to what they want from me?
➡ Do I know when the facility expects to make a decision? In other words, do I know how long I need to wait before knowing they do/do not expect to hire me?
➡ Do I know what follow-up is suggested? In other words, do I know if they will call me or send me a letter or if I am expected to call them?

by suggesting you view yourself as a professional and you make every attempt to keep your professional life separate from your private life. You may also wish to reassure him or her that you intend to devote as much time as necessary to be successful in your job.

To further prepare for the interview, Kief and Scheerer (2001) suggest participating in a mock interview. Some OT and OTA educational programs actually require their students to contact a local facility and set up a mock interview with an occupational therapy department director. This is a good way to role-play and practice for a real-life interview. The director may be asked to complete a feedback form on the student's performance (Kief & Scheerer, 2001), critiquing the student's professional behavior and interpersonal skills. University and college career services centers or placement offices also offer students the opportunity to participate in a mock interview to prepare for upcoming interviews. If you want to see what a potential employer might use to rate your performance in an interview, refer to *Applicant Interview Analysis* (p. 187) and *Things You Should Not Do In the Interview* (p. 188).

AFTER THE INTERVIEW

Send a thank-you note within 1 day of the interview to each person who has participated in interviewing you, such as the human resources person, the occupational therapy manager, and the collective group of therapists who may have spent time with you. This thank-you note must be handwritten or word-processed. Never send thank-you notes by e-mail or use electronic cards (see *Answers to Questions Students Often Ask* on p. 188).

REFERENCES

Adams, B. (2001). *The everything job interview book.* Holbrook, MA: Adams Media.

Dorio, M. (2000). *The complete idiot's guide to the perfect interview.* Indianapolis, IN: Alpha Books.

Drafke, M. (1994). *Working in health care.* Philadelphia, PA: F. A. Davis.

Fox, J. J. (2001). *Don't send a résumé.* New York, NY: Hyperion.

APPLICANT INTERVIEW ANALYSIS

Name of Applicant:
Date of Interview:
Time of Interview:
Candidate for:
Please report your interview impressions by checking the one most appropriate box in each area.

1. Appearance
- ○   Untidy.
- ○   Somewhat careless about personal appearance.
- ○   Satisfactory personal appearance.
- ○   Better than average appearance.

2. Personality
- ○   Appears very distant and aloof.
- ○   Approachable; fairly friendly.
- ○   Warm; friendly; sociable.
- ○   Very sociable and outgoing.

3. Poise-Stability
- ○   Ill at ease; is "jumpy" and appears nervous.
- ○   Somewhat tense; is easily irritated.
- ○   About as poised as the average person.
- ○   Sure of self; well composed.

4. Communication Ability
- ○   Expresses self poorly.
- ○   Does less than average job at expressing self.
- ○   Average fluency and expression.
- ○   Communicates well.

5. Alertness
- ○   Appears slow to "catch on."
- ○   Appears rather slow; requires more than average explanation.
- ○   Appears to grasp ideas with average ability.
- ○   Appears quick to understand; perceives very well.

6. Knowledge of Field
- ○   Appears to have poor knowledge of field.
- ○   Appears to have some knowledge of field.
- ○   An average amount of knowledge is demonstrated.
- ○   Appears to have excellent knowledge of field.

7. Experience in Field
- ○   No relationship between applicant's background and job requirements.
- ○   Fair relationship between applicant's background and job requirements.
- ○   Average amount of meaningful background and experience.
- ○   Excellent background; considerable experience in the field.

8. Drive
- ○   Appears to have poorly defined skills.
- ○   Appears to set goals too low.
- ○   Appears to have average goals.
- ○   Appears to have high desire to achieve.

9. Overall
- ○   Definitely unsatisfactory candidate.
- ○   Substandard candidate.
- ○   Average candidate.
- ○   Definitely above average candidate.
- ○   Outstanding candidate.

APPLICANT INTERVIEW ANALYSIS (CONTINUED)

This applicant should be considered further   ◯   Yes   ◯   No   If no, state reason:

If YES, request reference check   ◯   Yes   ◯   No
If NO, would you recommend consideration at future date for this or any other position?
◯   Yes   ◯   No   Remarks:

Additional comments:

Salary Quote: Start Date: Status:

Return completed form to human resources

Reprinted with permission from Healthsouth Harmarville Rehabilitation Hospital, Pittsburgh, PA.

THINGS YOU SHOULD NOT DO IN THE INTERVIEW

➡ Watch the clock.
➡ Eat, drink, chew gum, smoke.
➡ Try to be funny.
➡ Be aloof.
➡ Appear overly concerned about money.
➡ Take extraneous or copious notes; however, taking brief notes may be acceptable. The manager may actually be impressed with your perceived thoroughness.

ANSWERS TO QUESTIONS STUDENTS OFTEN ASK

➡ When should I start looking for a job?
Approximately 3 to 4 months before you really want to start working. Many students start their search in the brief time they have between fieldwork rotations or at the start of their last level II fieldwork experience.
➡ Where do I find out about jobs?
See the section on "Finding Places to Send Your Résumé or Call for an Interview."
➡ When do I send out my résumé?
In accordance with the time frame mentioned above, as soon as you find a place that is of interest to you, send a résumé. Many students send out resumes while still on their last level II fieldwork experience. This may give them an advantage in becoming employed immediately upon completion of fieldwork. It also means they will receive their first paycheck sooner. If you have student loans that are going to require attention as soon as you are no longer considered a college student, obtaining gainful employment may be a looming source of stress.
➡ Where do I send my résumé?
Again, see "Finding Places to Send Your Résumé or Call for an Interview."
➡ What should I say in the cover letter?
Go back and read the previous section, titled "Writing the Cover Letter."
➡ What should I do if I do not hear back from a place where my résumé was sent?
Call to make sure it was received and to let the facility know you are interested in talking to them further.

Gilfoyle, E., & Christiansen, C. (1987). Research: The quest for truth and the key to excellence. *Am J Occup Ther, 41,* 7-8.

Jackson, T., & Jackson, E. (1996). *The new perfect résumé.* New York, NY: Doubleday.

Kief, C., & Scheerer, C. (2001). *Clinical competencies in occupational therapy.* Upper Saddle River, NJ: Prentice Hall.

Chapter 17

Professional Development

Karen Sladyk, PhD, OTR, FAOTA

You worked so hard to finish your OT or OTA program, and celebrations are required, but those who think education is finally done are gypping themselves and their clients. Learning is lifelong. Those who participate in learning throughout their lives also report greater satisfaction and wellness in their personal lives.

All new grads experience transition issues as they begin work. It is not uncommon to feel both an expert and a total novice at the same time. Occupational therapy education has provided you with the skills to be a competent entry-level practitioner (Accreditation Council for Occupational Therapy Education [ACOTE], 1998a, 1998b), yet competency is an ongoing set of skills (American Occupational Therapy Association [AOTA], 1995). Professional development should be a lifelong dynamic goal for all occupational therapy practitioners, yet some people allow themselves to stagnate and make excuses for failing to grow professionally. Make it your goal not to be one of those practitioners who stopped professional growth soon after school.

This chapter is designed to show readers the wealth of professional education opportunities available to them. By the end of the chapter, you will understand the following:

➡ The value of membership in professional organizations.

➡ How to set long- and short-term professional advancement goals.

➡ The formal and informal methods to develop professional knowledge.

➡ How to self-appraise skills and develop an action plan.

AOTA Membership: The Easiest Professional Development Plan

As an occupational therapy educator, I am often called to answer questions about the profession. The answer is usually a very simple referral to AOTA for the documents the person needs. Unfortunately, about half the time, the practitioner says he or she is not a member of AOTA. When I ask why not, the answer is usually money or that he or she forgot to renew. AOTA, like all other membership organizations, serves its members. Nonmember OT practitioners sometime become upset when AOTA will not serve them as well. I always ask, would you expect any other organization to serve you if you were not a member? Can you walk into a social club and expect to be served lunch at members' prices? AOTA is a non-profit organization developed by its members to serve its members. It has a wealth of knowledge it is eager to share with members, including evidence-based practice, so if you forgot to renew your membership, call AOTA and join. If money is your justification, consider this trick I learned from my sister (see *What's Your Time Really Worth?* on p. 193).

Now, consider AOTA membership at approximately $200 per year. Divided by 365 days, that's less than 55 cents per day—half a can of soda pop. Now, consider just some of the benefits 55 cents per day gets you with AOTA: professionals who advocate for OT to Congress; professionals who fight Medicare when they want to cut reimbursements; professionals who work with states to keep occupational therapy practice from being invaded by other disciplines; a full occupational therapy library; a sleek web site; a place to post your résumé; a huge national OT conference; and access to numerous discounts on insurance, credit cards, and travel costs. Can you find anyone else to do all of this for you for 55 cents per day? I'm willing to pay 55 cents per day just to have the ear of Congress because that alone would cost me more in time and money if I tried to do that myself.

AOTA has a wealth of formal and informal professional development opportunities such as the journal *American Journal of Occupational Therapy (AJOT)*, the trade magazine *OT Practice*, numerous self-study programs, a national conference, special traveling regional conferences, the Wilma West Library, a foundation that supports research, a book and publication department, a web site with up-to-the-minute information, fax-on-demand services, and live people who answer your calls when you need information. Many of these professional development opportunities award certificates for state licensure or workplace requirements. AOTA (1995) has developed a self-appraisal booklet that can guide you in assessing your current skills and developing a professional development plan. In addition, AOTA is working with the national certification organization to collaborate on future professional development requirements for the profession.

Besides joining AOTA, consider joining your state occupational therapy association. This is a wonderful place to network and develop leadership skills through volunteering. AOTA can provide you with the state association membership contact person or check around at your school because applications are likely posted on a bulletin board.

Long- and Short-Term Professional Goals

Remember being asked, "What do you want to be when you grow up?" Well, here you are, an occupational therapy practitioner, and I'm asking the same question again. What occupations are in your life, and what occupations are future goals? Use the activity in *Organizing Goals* (p. 193) to help organize your plans, keeping in mind that they will change over time.

Notice that there is no attempt to separate personal from professional development. As we know from the study of occupation, no one role stands alone. A new graduate may have as a short-term goal to find a generalist entry-level position as an OT or OTA, but may also have plans to marry and start a family. Students occasionally tell me that they want a management position to better support their interests outside of work. Some students have told me they want to teach OT, understanding a teaching career means continuing college education.

The last question about other careers is intended to stimulate creative thinking. Career goals change over a lifetime because, when you grow, your career goals grow too (Ellis, 2000). Skills developed in an occupational therapy career are helpful in other careers. Many occupational therapy practitioners have opened their own businesses including play equipment, career coaching, craft supplies, and even a quilt shop in my hometown.

By reviewing your long- and short-term goals, you can begin to plan your professional development. A specific professional development plan will be the ladder to accomplishing your goals. Finding the right combination of educational opportunities becomes the foundation to your professional development.

WHAT'S YOUR TIME REALLY WORTH?

➡ Begin by writing down your current hourly rate of pay.
➡ After taxes, approximately what is your hourly rate of pay?
➡ Divide that in half.
➡ If you can pay anyone else to do something for you at this rate, hire him or her.

ORGANIZING GOALS

	Date:	Date:	Date:
List all of your current roles and occupations			
Where do you want to be in 1 year?			
What roles and occupations will you likely hold in 1 year?			
Where do you want to be in 5 years?			
What roles and occupations will you likely hold in 5 years?			
Where do you want to be in 10 years?			
What roles and occupations will you likely hold in 10 years?			
Besides OT, what other careers interest you?			

FORMAL VERSUS INFORMAL EDUCATION

What! More school? Think about what it is like when you go away on vacation. You eat all your favorite foods, do all kinds of fun stuff. Oddly, by the end of your vacation, you are looking forward to getting home. Once you are home, you wonder what it would be like to go back on vacation. While you are in school, the thought of more school does not sound appealing but you may feel differently later.

Formal education is typically a college degree or a formal organizational certificate, while informal education, often called *continuing education*, includes a variety of learning from having a mentor to attending a local conference. There are many experts in education who will argue that one type of education is better than another type. You will likely get advice on this topic even if you do not seek the advice. The ultimate opinion, of course, is yours. The bottom line is that you continue to educate yourself and stay current in your field. Before you form an opinion about formal edu-

cation versus informal continuing education, you should make sure you understand all the options available to you.

FORMAL PROFESSIONAL DEVELOPMENT OPPORTUNITIES

Formal education is less varied than informal education, but is generally more highly regarded by society as a valued educational experience. Typically, this includes college degrees and specialty certifications from recognized organizations. Although higher in costs and time commitments, formal education is easier to document gained knowledge because of the resulting degree or credential.

Traditional formal education means returning to a college or university to seek a higher degree than the one you currently possess. The benefits of another degree might include self-esteem, a promotion, a pay raise, and mastery of a subject (Peters, 1997). Some

OT Degree or Related Area

Question:	Yes	No
What are my goals in earning another degree?		
Where do I plan to be after the degree is done?		
Do I plan to continue to work at my current job?		
Is occupational therapy something I want to study more?		
Is there another area that will enhance my skills in OT?		
In what areas do I have interest?		
Do I want to be promoted to a higher skill level position?		
Do I want to teach occupational therapy?		

Adapted from Sladyk, K. (1997). Graduate school and continuing education. In K. Sladyk (Ed.), *OT student primer: A guide to college success* (pp. 323-329). Thorofare, NJ: SLACK Incorporated.

workplaces offer promotions or pay raises with another degree, while others do not. Many workplaces even encourage college study by offering special discounts, time off, or tuition reimbursement programs. If you think you are likely to return to college after you start working, be sure to check into tuition assistance programs with the personnel department when you interview.

As you likely know, college degrees are offered in four levels: associate, bachelor, masters, and doctorate. Traditionally, the first three levels of degrees are focused in either the arts or sciences. Some schools offer specialty degrees, such as masters in Occupational Therapy (MOT) or masters in Social Work (MSW). Traditionally, the doctoral level is a PhD, a research-focused doctoral degree. Other doctoral-level degrees are now available, such as an EdD (education), ScD (science), JD (law), and new programs emerging in occupational therapy called the Clinical Doctorate. Each type of degree has different requirements, and each school can design the degree as it feels necessary within the laws of the state. Generally, each degree requires the following as minimums: associate—60 credit hours; bachelor—120 credit hours; masters—36 credit hours above a bachelor degree; doctorate—varies greatly depending on degree.

OTA programs are usually at the associate level, and OT programs are bachelor or masters level.

Beginning in January 2007, bachelor degree OT programs will no longer be accredited, resulting in all current entry-level OT programs converting to graduate education. Because of this change, students with a masters degree in entry-level practice may be interested in a second masters degree in advanced practice occupational therapy.

Deciding to go back to college for education beyond your entry-level degree in OTA or OT means evaluating your interests and career goals. You will have to decide if you want a degree in occupational therapy or if you want a degree in a related area. The decision should be based on your needs and goals. Only you can evaluate what area of study you want to pursue. Consider your interests and long-term plans. Discuss your thoughts with people who have done what you are thinking about. Use *OT Degree or Related Area* to stimulate your thinking.

You may be lucky enough to be able to pack up and move to another area to go to school full-time, but more than likely, your viable degree choices will be limited by several factors. These include drivable distance from your home, being within your budget and the tuition reimbursement rules of work, being willing to take part-time students, being flexible to fit into your schedule, including your family's schedule.

Almost every school has at least an abbreviated catalog on its web site, so the traditional way of calling schools and requesting a catalog is now old fash-

AREAS OF STUDY

Occupational Therapy
➡ OTA to OT programs
➡ Advance practice masters with focus in developmental disabilities, mental health, physical rehabilitation, management, education, research, or occupational science
➡ Doctoral programs specific to OT

Related Areas
➡ Adult learning
➡ Community health
➡ Counseling
➡ Education
➡ Information management
➡ Health care management
➡ Human resources
➡ Law
➡ Management
➡ Marriage and family
➡ Neuroscience or movement
➡ Psychology or forensics
➡ Public health
➡ Rehabilitation
➡ Social work

Adapted from Sladyk, K. (1997). Graduate school and continuing education. In K. Sladyk (Ed.), *OT student primer: A guide to college success* (pp. 323-329). Thorofare, NJ: SLACK Incorporated.

---

ioned. Web sites typically have virtual campus tours and student testimonials that can provide you with information about the college; however, remember that a web site is really only an advertisement. Screen possible schools by talking with people in your community. Once you view the catalogs, look for programs of interest. Consider the tuition costs and what you can afford.

The choices of possible degrees for the OTA or OT are endless, but you may be restricted by a geographical area. If so, the best way to find a degree that interests you is to review local college catalogs. If your local community or college library is large enough, you may find a section of all the local colleges' catalogs. This can save you time over using the Internet and allows you to compare aspects side by side. Some of the popular areas of study for OTAs and OTs are included in *Areas of Study*.

When you have decided which program is for you, complete the application and apply. Some schools at the masters and doctorate level require scholastic tests, such as the Graduate Record Exam (GRE). Several different exams are available, but the GRE is the most common. The GRE is similar to the SAT you took in high school. Although taking the GRE is no walk in the park, it will not be nearly as bad as you remember the SAT. The key is being prepared and reviewing before the test using software or study manuals from your local bookstore. Do not take the GRE cold, without preparation. You can take the GRE as many times as you want, but all of your scores are reported until the score becomes 5 years old and is dropped from the record, so bad results can follow you for 5 years.

OTA to OT Programs

In the past, OTAs have been frustrated because national rules about transferring OTA classes did not allow OT credit; however, with entry-level OT practice changing to masters degree, an interesting thing is happening for OTAs wishing to become OTs. Many colleges are now accepting OTA classes into liberal arts bachelor degree programs leading to a masters in entry-level OT. This means that the OTA is no longer losing a year of credits and is spending the same amount of time in school but finishing with a masters degree instead of a bachelor degree.

OTAs should not feel the need to move to an OT degree. Keep in mind that the profession supports both OTAs and OTs, and there is never any assumption that OTAs must work to become OTs. When an OTA does wish to become an OT, AOTA can provide a list of special programs specific to this audience.

Advance Practice Masters Degrees

The practicing OT, either bachelor or entry-level masters degree, will have to decide if an advanced masters in occupational therapy is his or her preference or a masters in a related area. Most OTs earning masters in the past had little choice. masters degrees in occupational therapy were fairly rare. This has changed, and many schools offer advanced degrees to OTs. Many advanced degrees allow students to specialize in an area of interest such as developmental disabilities, pediatric, or management. Some degrees focus on education or research. If you are interested in an advanced degree in occupational therapy, request a catalog or visit the web site to review the program. If the program looks of interest, call the school and ask to speak to a student in the program. The student should be able to address your questions on pace, schedule, requirements, teachers, and content of classes. You may be able to sit in on a class or attend an open house.

Doctoral Degrees

At this time, you may be thinking, "Is she crazy?" I know the doctoral idea is not appealing to a lot of you, but there are a few who have been hiding this thought in the backs of their minds. Doctoral level work is most certainly a challenge, but a challenge at which many OTs have succeeded. If you hold as your goal a faculty appointment or advance practice in a leading institution, doctoral level education is highly desirable.

Just like the masters degrees mentioned above, doctorates can be in occupational therapy or a related area. Several universities offer doctoral education in OT, and some contain online classes that limit required time on campus. For those interested in other related areas, it is possible to combine your love of OT with a new study area. For example, most doctoral programs will allow you to transfer in up to two classes. Most will allow independent studies. So if you are an OT studying adult learning, you may be able to transfer a class in clinical reasoning and a class on fieldwork into your program. An independent study can compare and contrast clinical reasoning with theories on critical thinking in adulthood. Lastly, you can use occupational therapy as a component of your dissertation. Check with the doctoral program you are interested in for its rules and regulations.

If you think a doctorate is in your future, consider looking at combination programs that give you a masters degree on your way to your doctorate. Also, carefully weigh the benefits of a PhD, ScD, EdD, or clinical doctorate. Each has its own benefits. Although all require great disciplined study, the PhD has a long history of being well established and is often privately acknowledged as the preferred degree. Lastly, understand the program requirements before you start. Will you be required to do a full-time residency? Can you take classes part-time? How is the research component of the degree managed? The more you know before you start, the easier it will be to finish.

Specialty Certifications

Many professional organizations, including AOTA, offer specialty certificates. Some organizations provide intensive education followed by testing to gain certification, such as NDT or SI training. Other organizations provide strict qualification requirements followed by testing to gain credentials, such as "board certified in..." Each organization can provide you with the requirements of the certification. Having the requirements in mind well before you qualify can help design your professional development plan to prepare you for future certifications.

INFORMAL PROFESSIONAL DEVELOPMENT OPPORTUNITIES

All this discussion about formal education may have your head spinning. Informal professional development opportunities might better meet your current needs. Continuing education has seen an explosion of ideas in occupational therapy recently. Pick up any occupational therapy trade magazine and you will find pages of educational opportunities. Not only are conferences listed, but AOTA offers members self-study programs, online computer education, and a national occupational therapy conference that attracts 5,000 people at one time. There is no limit to conference topics. Many occupational therapy practitioners favor traditional conferences for continuing education, but informal learning can take many forms (see *Opportunities for Professional Development in Informal Educational Experiences* on p. 197).

An important aspect of any educational experience is not just participating, but the resulting knowledge

OPPORTUNITIES FOR PROFESSIONAL DEVELOPMENT IN INFORMAL EDUCATIONAL EXPERIENCES

➡ *AJOT*, SIS newsletters, *OT Practice* magazine
➡ AOTA annual conference
➡ Asking an expert at work to mentor you
➡ Internet sources listed in Appendix B
➡ New books recently published
➡ Online computer conference and online practice support
➡ Participating in peer review
➡ Participating in research projects
➡ Reviewing journals for evidence-based practice
➡ Self-study programs
➡ State OT association conferences
➡ Supervising level I or II students
➡ Volunteering to present a topic
➡ Work performance review
➡ Workplace in-services or journal clubs
➡ Workshops or seminars
➡ Writing for publication

being used effectively in your practice (Hinojosa et al., 2000). Documenting knowledge gained from informal education is more difficult than formal education, but is equally important. Consider demonstrating your continuing competence through attendance certificates, examinations, work performance reviews, peer reviews, summative papers or presentations, or a professional portfolio as outlined in Chapter 15.

Many occupational therapy schools offer free or inexpensive conferences related to educational issues, such as fieldwork. These conferences allow attendees to enjoy the latest information about education at a greatly reduced price. In addition, OTs can share experiences and educational models that are effective in the clinic. Sometimes, occupational therapy schools offer certificates of advanced training. When you take a cluster of four masters level classes, you earn the certificate. Those interested in continuing on to an advanced degree can count the certificate classes toward a masters degree.

Online classes or self-study programs allow OTAs and OTs to study a topic at their own pace without leaving their homes or workplaces. These self-contained conferences award certificates of completion, and some can be accepted for masters degree credits. With these types of continuing education opportunities, rural OTAs and OTs can participate without leaving home. Self-study programs can be done in a small group, allowing for questions and feedback, as well as networking. Other online services are available from AOTA, including resources for help on special problems.

Many individual and specialty groups also offer conferences. You will find these listed in the occupational therapy trade magazines. Fees for these conferences vary greatly, and the topics are usually specific with some advanced skills required. The best way to stay up-to-date on these specialty topics is to scan the conference listings regularly.

Many continuing education opportunities are mailed directly to your home. The *American Journal of Occupational Therapy* (*AJOT*) provides you with monthly, up-to-date research in occupational therapy. The level of writing sometimes intimidates readers, but the editor and reviewers work hard to make the articles clear. The more you read the journal, the more you will understand. One way to better understand journal articles is to first read about evidence-based practice concepts. Check your college textbooks for an introduction to evidence-based practice. Understanding these foundation skills will be helpful when reading the articles.

AJOT makes an excellent continuing education opportunity because it is delivered to you, is self-paced, and is available at no additional cost with your membership. *OT Practice* magazine provides a more informal continuing education opportunity by focusing on current practice in a practical format. Like *AJOT*, it comes right to your home and is included with your AOTA membership. Often, *OT Practice* has self-study units included in the magazine. Read the self-study article, take a short multiple-choice test, pay a small fee, and get continuing education credit.

TRUE CASE EXAMPLES

April has known for years that she would like an academic career long-term, but first she must finish college and become a practitioner. She has carefully watched her faculty while in class and wants to position herself for an educational position further in her career. She has done a lot of research about the process, including skimming books on the topic at her college library. She has not shared much of this information with her peers, but a good friend suggested she talk to a faculty member if she is serious about this. April is a bit apprehensive because she knows she is not one of the "best" students in class and is afraid the faculty may think her long-term goal is out of touch considering she has not even graduated yet. During class, the faculty member discusses professional development issues in her state. April takes the opportunity to address the issue after class. The faculty member meets with her and listens to what she already knows about academia. Together, they set up an action plan that includes graduation, experience, supervising fieldwork students, graduate school, teaching part-time, and other experiences that can position her for an academic job in a time-effective manner.

Blake is a recent graduate with about 9 months of experience in general physical rehabilitation. He works for a for-profit contracting company that has a strong ethical code that is attractive to Blake. He sees that the company is growing, and he is interested in staying with the company as it grows. Blake mentions this during supervision, and the supervisor explains how she became a department director. The supervisor suggests that Blake talk to the regional director the next time she is visiting the site. The regional director explains what the corporate office looks for when hiring managers and suggests Blake consider returning to school part-time or attending management conferences. The regional director also suggests that Blake consider supervising a level II student as he becomes qualified to see if he enjoys supervising others. At the next supervision meeting with his department director, the two outline a professional development plan that moves Blake toward management experience.

Lauren has 5 years of experience in mental health, working in a state psychiatric hospital. She really enjoys working with the patients but has found that she misses the conversations she used to have with peers while in school. Lauren is not sure what she wants to do in the long-term. She enjoys supervising level II students and directing a small subdivision of the rehabilitation department. She wants to pursue an additional degree, but one that has flexibility for future planning. She develops her own action plan to investigate degrees from several colleges in driving distance. While reading the catalogs, she finds one that perfectly meets her needs and fits her limited budget.

Seth has 20 years of experience as a school-based occupational therapy practitioner. He has concentrated all his professional development in conferences related to children from birth to age 5. He is considered a statewide leader in this area. Now, he is interested in sharing this knowledge and applies for a tenure-track position at a local community college. He is disappointed when he does not get the position, which goes to someone with less experience. Seth asks for feedback and discovers that his extensive list of specialty training worked against him because the interviewing team felt his focus was too narrow. Although there had been numerous free conferences sponsored by the local college consortium concerning more general practice topics, Seth had never attended anything outside of his specialty. The interviewing team recognized his expertise but wanted someone who was an expert and up-to-date on general occupational therapy issues as well. Seth redesigned his professional development plan to include other occupational therapy issues and found that these conferences gave him additional insights into his specialty area. He was more confident sharing his knowledge at conferences because he had a renewed foundation that he shared with others outside of his specialty.

SELF-APPRAISAL AND ACTION PLAN

Now that the chapter has addressed the endless professional development opportunities available for OT practitioners, you need to develop an action plan that specifically addresses your needs. While it is fine to attend conferences in your specialty area, consider reviewing your long-term goals before signing up for another conference. Will you always be employed in your current practice area? Is management, specialty, or education a future goal? Are you looking to focus all your energy into a specific practice area? Read *True Case Examples*.

Once you have your professional development action plan clear, how will you document your skills so you can show potential future employers? Review the chapters on résumés and portfolios to develop your own documentation system. Remember, it is much easier to keep these tools updated than to wait until a new job opportunity presents itself, and you scurry through your home looking for that forgotten certificate.

SUMMARY

It is your professional responsibility to stay current in the practice of occupational therapy because it is important to your consumers of occupational therapy. Furthering your education can take two different roads. First, formal education such as returning to a college or university for another degree can develop or refine skills. Second, less formal continuing education allows the learner to be specific in his or her learning needs. Educational experts disagree as to which type is best. The learner must evaluate his or her own needs and then establish a professional development action plan specific to those needs.

REFERENCES

Accreditation Council for Occupational Therapy Education. (1998a). *Standards for an accredited educational program for the occupational therapist.* Bethesda, MD: American Occupational Therapy Association.

Accreditation Council for Occupational Therapy Education. (1998b). *Standards for an accredited educational program for the occupational therapist assistant.* Bethesda, MD: American Occupational Therapy Association.

American Occupational Therapy Association. (1995). *Developing, maintaining, and updating competency in occupational therapy: A guide to self-appraisal.* Bethesda, MD: Author.

Ellis, D. (2000). *Becoming a master student.* Boston, MA: Houghton Mifflin Company.

Hinojosa, J., Bowen, R., Case-Smith, J., Epstein, C., Moyers, P., & Schwope, C. (2000). Self-initiated continuing competence. *OT Practice, December,* CE1-CE8.

Peters, R. L. (1997). *Getting what you came for: The smart student's guide to earning a masters or a PhD.* New York, NY: The Noonday Press.

Sladyk, K. (1997). Graduate school and continuing education. In K. Sladyk (Ed.), *OT student primer: A guide to college success* (pp. 323-329). Thorofare, NJ: SLACK Incorporated.

Chapter 18

SUPERVISING YOUR OWN STUDENTS

Karen Sladyk, PhD, OTR, FAOTA

Supervising your own level I and II students is an excellent way to update your skills, provide service to your profession, and help a novice practitioner grow into a professional. Although a serious and demanding task, many supports and resources are available for supervising fieldwork students. By the end of this chapter, you will do the following:

➠ Dispel myths concerning fieldwork.

➠ Understand the stakeholder's perspective on the fieldwork experience.

➠ Be able to develop a level I and II fieldwork program at his or her site.

➠ Be able to use strategies to assist failing students.

You understand the basic concepts of fieldwork because every OT or OTA experienced fieldwork as part of his or her program. You just need some help getting started. First, let's examine some myths about fieldwork programs.

MYTHS CONCERNING FIELDWORK

➡ A good fieldwork experience is one in physical disability and one in mental health.

➡ OTAs cannot supervise fieldwork students.

➡ The supervising OT or OTA should be full-time in one site.

➡ Pediatric or other specialties should be saved for a third level II.

➡ Supervising students takes too much time.

➡ Too much revenue is lost if students are in a physical rehabilitation setting.

➡ The best supervision model is one student to one OT.

And now, the realities of today's occupational therapy practice. As you know, what we held as traditional occupational therapy practice has seen dramatic changes recently. When fieldwork sites were in extreme shortages in the early 1990s, OT schools began to experiment with *nontraditional* fieldwork sites. Now routinely called *emerging practice areas*, occupational therapy has seen these new areas become *traditional* sites for practitioners. Although many OT practitioners are still employed in hospitals, rehabilitation programs, and public schools, many more are in innovating sites that they have developed themselves. Students in OT and OTA programs are learning that emerging practice areas provide exciting, flexible, and challenging opportunities to practice. Let us briefly look at the myths again.

A Good Fieldwork Experience is One in Physical Disability and One in Mental Health

The Accreditation Council for Occupational Therapy Education (ACOTE) (1998a, 1998b) states that fieldwork must be across the disciplines and with a variety of ages. Because many OT and OTA programs do not even separate their curriculum into physical disabilities and mental health any more, fieldwork is not divided either. Because good occupational therapy means treating the whole person, any site that has OT is an appropriate fieldwork site.

OTAs Cannot Supervise Fieldwork Students

ACOTE (1998a, 1998b) allows for an OTA to supervise both level I and II students. As with any

responsibility, the OTA's skills should be considered, and typically level II supervision is done in collaboration with an OT.

The Supervising OT or OTA Should be Full-Time in One Site

Initially thought to be true and then seen as a luxury, this myth just is not the reality of today's practice. Level I and II fieldwork introduces the student to the profession. If a supervising practitioner is not full-time or not in one site, then that is what current practice entails. Students should not be hidden from these experiences.

Pediatric or Other Specialties Should Be Saved for a Third Level II

Specialty practices may have specific needs when accepting a student, but because today's practice includes these disciplines, students should participate. Because students come to the profession with a variety of skills, specialized practice centers may find interviews helpful in finding students prepared to accept the challenge of a special fieldwork site.

Supervising Students Takes Too Much Time

Initially, especially the first week or so, students do take a lot of time. This extra time in the beginning likely benefits the supervisor in the last weeks, when a student is independent and frees the supervisor to tackle other tasks like the QA report that is overdue. Later in this chapter, supervision techniques are addressed further.

Too Much Revenue is Lost if Students are in a Physical Rehabilitation Setting

Medicare has made recent rulings that have limited students from billing for some of their services. However, this has not totally limited all student services. For example, to accept Medicare reimbursement for some patients, the facility must agree to service all patients without regard to reimbursement generated. Once skills are established, students can service consumers who do not qualify for reimbursement.

The Best Supervision Model is One Student to One OT

Once again, this is a luxury of a slower-paced practice of the past. This type of fieldwork model may not only be ineffective, but a time waster, too. Research (Declute & Ladyshewsky, 1993; Hengel & Romeo, 1995) suggests two students to one supervisor results in students working problems out together instead of always asking the supervisor. In addition, two students together have someone to talk with during down time such as lunch, freeing the supervisor from having a student always with him or her.

MAJOR PLAYERS IN FIELDWORK

As with every experience, there are major players or stakeholders in the fieldwork experience. Clearly, the student is a stakeholder, but this section focuses on the roles of others, including ACOTE, which maintains the rules on fieldwork, the school, and the fieldwork site. Each group has its own concerns and rules it must follow. Each group holds a slightly different perspective on fieldwork.

ACOTE (1998a, 1998b) has developed the standards that all OT and OTA programs must follow to hold accreditation and have their students eligible to take the practice examination. ACOTE established these rules to ensure graduates are competent to practice OT. The standards state that all schools must have level I and II fieldwork experiences and that these experiences must be integrated into the curriculum. ACOTE further expects the schools to collaborate with fieldwork sites and to document this collaboration in detail. Each school has a different way of addressing these standards, but likely this falls mainly to one faculty member, the academic fieldwork coordinator (AFWC) of the school. The AFWC is likely the first person you will contact if you are interested in supervising a fieldwork student.

The AFWC at any school will have a system in place to get your facility set up to have level I and II fieldwork students. The AFWC will ask many questions concerning your facility, establish a contract that outlines expectations and protections, and set up a site visit. Further, the AFWC will ask for a contact person that he or she should call in the future. If the department is large and has several staff who might be assigned a student, the department may want to assign organizational duties to the department head or a clinical education coordinator. The initial contact with the AFWC should provide you with opportunities to have all your questions answered.

Because a fieldwork site will have some legal responsibilities, the site's administration should be involved from the initial contact. As supervising students is not unique to occupational therapy, administration is likely familiar with the procedure and will be supportive. If the department is asked to provide evidence that fieldwork has benefits for the facility, use the review in *Research Supporting the Benefits of Accepting Fieldwork Students* (p. 204). Demonstrating how fieldwork fits into the facility's mission statement and philosophy can also help reluctant administrators understand the benefits of accepting students.

DEVELOPING A FIELDWORK PROGRAM SPECIFIC TO YOUR SITE

Once you have made initial contact with a school and have the contract process moving forward, it is time to start developing a plan to accept your first students. Where you start in the plan depends on the resources available to you. The AFWC with whom you are working might be able to provide you with sample fieldwork programs or you can network with other practitioners who have fieldwork programs in place. A generic checklist outline for level II fieldwork is provided here and is briefly summarized in *Establishing a Level II Fieldwork* (p. 204).

To begin, gather a committee of OT practitioners who might be interested in fieldwork, or assign one person to develop a program.

Establish a brief list of basic skills required of an entry-level practitioner at your site. Job descriptions and essential requirement lists might be helpful. Decide if an initial interview is required by your facility before a student is accepted or if students can be assigned to the site in consultation with the AFWC. Preacceptance interviews must follow the same procedures as employment interviews. Questions must be limited to accepted employment procedure and cannot include personal or health questions. Also gather any policies that require health-screening information, such as inoculations, and decide how much, if any, sick time a student can have during fieldwork.

If you are a member of the American Occupational Therapy Association (AOTA), visit the web site (www.aota.org) for additional supportive information concerning fieldwork. Also consider completing AOTA's *Meeting the Fieldwork Challenge Self-Study Program* (Merrill & Crist, 2000). Although the program is expensive to purchase, the AFWC at your local school may be able to lend the program to you at no charge.

RESEARCH SUPPORTING THE BENEFITS OF ACCEPTING FIELDWORK STUDENTS

Forming positive professional attitudes
➡ Atwater & Davis. (1990). Fieldwork in mental health changes student's attitudes.
➡ Swinehart & Meyers. (1992). Outcomes are affected by different expectations.
➡ Lyons & Ziviani. (1995). Benefits of community-based practice.
➡ Tompson & Ryan. (1996). Role of fieldwork on professional socialization.

Fits facility purpose and goals
➡ Kautzmann. (1987). Describes how schools and facilities see level I goals.

Cost benefits
➡ Meyers. (1995). Describes how to minimize costs and maximize benefits.
➡ Shalik. (1987). Level II fieldwork students generally result in positive revenue.
➡ Shalik & Shalik. (1988). Most level II fieldwork in physical rehabilitation or mental health results in positive revenue for the facility.

Recruitment and retention of staff
➡ Hischmann. (1990). Fieldwork benefits on recruitment and retention of staff.

Flexible models addressing staff shortages
➡ Adelstein, Cohn, Baker, & Barnes. (1990). Part-time level II fieldwork.
➡ Siebert. (1997). Home care fieldwork program.

Educational benefits
➡ Walker. (1995). Joint collaborative projects benefit all.
➡ Bloomer. (1995). Applied research during fieldwork benefits facility.

ESTABLISHING A LEVEL II FIELDWORK

➡ Gather people interested in developing fieldwork.

➡ Establish a list of basic skills required of an entry-level practitioner at your site.

➡ Visit www.aota.org for additional supportive information concerning fieldwork.

➡ Gather the evaluation forms local colleges use to evaluate students.

➡ Write specific behavioral objectives for each item evaluated.

➡ Establish a supervision model.

➡ Decide how feedback will be provided.

➡ Decide how to assign consumers to the student with a timeline, including additional assignments.

➡ Write any policies or procedures related to students, add to department manual.

➡ Develop a student manual or consider having students develop one.

➡ Return any fieldwork forms sent by the AFWC.

➡ Evaluate the student experience considering all stakeholders.

Gather the evaluation forms local colleges use to evaluate students. Typically, this is AOTA's 1987 Fieldwork Evaluation (FWE), currently under revision.

Review the student evaluation forms, and write specific behavioral objectives for each item scored. This is a time-consuming task, and your AFWC may have samples from other programs to share with you. The time invested in making clear objectives will be greatly rewarded if you should later have a student who is not passing. Have peers review the fieldwork expectations. See *Sample Fieldwork Objectives* (p. 205) for sample student objectives.

SAMPLE FIELDWORK OBJECTIVES

➡ Gathers necessary information before assessment.
Performance: Reads referral.
Judgment: Checks with non-OT staff in professional manner.
Attitude: Shows eagerness to complete assessment.

➡ Establishes relevant long-term goals.
Performance: Writes measurable goals.
Judgment: Writes meaningful goals.
Attitude: Involves client in goal development.

➡ Contributes to discussions.
Performance: Plans with other OT students.
Judgment: Suggests activities meaningful to clients.
Attitude: Carries fair share of work.

➡ Demonstrates understanding of costs.
Performance: Seeks low-cost activities that are meaningful to clients with limited funds.
Judgment: Always considers cost when dealing with client's limited means.
Attitude: Never boasts of personal activities clearly above limited resources of clients.

Establish a supervision model to use. Although traditional supervision has meant one supervisor to one student, consider staffing at your facility. Multiple supervisors mean more time required for collaboration between supervisors; however, each supervisor is not responsible for the student's total experience. The thought of two students with one supervisor might sound exhausting, but this model has several time and energy benefits. First, the supervisor is freed of many of the "unofficial" duties of fieldwork. A pair of students can consult with each other before bringing treatment ideas and draft documentation notes to the supervisor. The students can eat lunch together or take breaks together, allowing the supervisor to address other issues without a student "in tow." A pair of students can tackle assignments together, resulting in higher quality products. In addition, a pair of students keeps a check on professional behaviors as the weaker student typically rises to the level of the stronger student. Confidence is stronger in a pair, and students seem to "jump right in" faster. Pairs of students are more productive earlier in their fieldwork. If you are going to explain the fire evacuation procedures to one, a second student listening does not add extra work. As for treatment supervision, the pair can treat together until the supervisor is confident they can begin treating alone.

Decide how feedback will be provided. Formal supervision meetings on a weekly basis can provide students with opportunities to discuss issues and problems. Although time consuming, these meetings also allow the supervisor to ask probing questions, coach, and evaluate clinical reasoning skills on a regular basis. If necessary, formal meetings are easier to document. This is especially helpful for a student who may not be passing. Even with an excellent student who is receiving informal feedback throughout the day, formal meetings are recommended at midterm and final evaluation.

Decide how to assign consumers to the student with a timeline working up to a full caseload by the last few weeks of the fieldwork assignment. Add to the timeline any additional assignments you want students to complete. Although it is traditional to have assignments such as case studies or in-services given to students, research into the type and number of assignments should be considered. Sladyk & Sheckley (2000) found that, as the number of student assignments increased over four, the more likely a student was to show a decline in clinical reasoning skills. The theory is that too many additional assignments kept students from developing solid thinking skills because they were busy finishing assignments. Consistently the most powerful activity identified by good clinical reasoning students was "really getting to know the patient as a person." When developing additional assignments, consider activities that benefit the student, the staff, and the consumer, as outlined in *Suggested Fieldwork*

SUGGESTED FIELDWORK ASSIGNMENTS THAT BENEFIT SEVERAL STAKEHOLDERS

➡ Allow students to closely follow several consumers, asking them to spend extra time to get to know them well.

➡ Develop a piece of equipment that can be used in assessment or treatment.

➡ Collect or analyze data for quality-assurance reports.

➡ Develop a consumer pamphlet for postdischarge information or home care programs.

➡ Plan activities that educate others in the facility about occupational therapy.

➡ Present an in-service on a new technique or frame of reference learned in school.

➡ Develop an educational resource file for staff and consumers.

➡ Complete a needs assessment to evaluate the potential for a new program.

➡ Develop an activity card file in an area of interest not currently covered in the facility.

Assignments that Benefit Several Stakeholders. Also consider how much "homework" time is expected of a student outside of fieldwork hours. It is acceptable to expect students to do additional assignments outside of fieldwork.

Write any policies or procedures that need to be included in your department manual concerning students in the practice. Gather any policy and procedure information or forms a student will need to know, and begin to develop a student manual.

Continue gathering material you feel is appropriate to share with students in a student manual. This may include orientation forms, assessment and treatment ideas, consumer handouts used by the department, examples of ideas for student assignments, documentation aids, or helpful outlines.

Return any fieldwork forms sent by the AFWC, including program descriptions, contact person, signed contracts, photocopy of your objectives, and fieldwork requirements for health and/or acceptance interviews. Some schools may ask you to hold a fieldwork slot as a "reservation" for the school. Decide how the department will manage numerous reservations or several students requesting the same dates.

Establish a method for evaluating the student experience considering all stakeholders.

Now that you have your fieldwork program in place, try it out with a student, and make adjustments as needed. Facilities will soon find that having students around improves everyone's performance and professional development. Successful students add to the facility and provide opportunities to evaluate potential employees, reducing advertising costs and retention issues.

THE UNSUCCESSFUL FIELDWORK STUDENT

There is no single fieldwork task harder than failing a student. As the gatekeeper of the profession, a heavy load is placed on the fieldwork supervisor, especially if terminating a student from a fieldwork. A cognitive and affective task, failing a student often means a disrupted occupational therapy practice and an exhausted supervisor.

There are many different reasons why students find themselves "in trouble" on fieldwork (Gutman, McCreedy, & Heisler, 1998). Most reasons can be summarized using the FWE. Performance typically involves the student not applying knowledge learned in school. Attitude includes failing to make changes after feedback, poor professional skills, poor time management skills, and not using professional development opportunities. Judgment involves safety, patient priorities, professional behavior, and problem solving. Other issues can include physical and emotional health problems.

Although a fieldwork supervisor may be asking, "How could the school let someone out like this?", the answer is often complex. Many students are successful in school because OT classes are very structured and the campus is student-centered. Problems often arise when the student moves from an environment centered around students to an environment centered around the OT consumer. This may trigger issues that did not show in the classroom. In addition, students with disabilities may have chosen not to disclose a disability that might have an effect on fieldwork perform-

LEARNING CONTRACT OPTIONS

Student:
   Review content specific to weaknesses
➡ Adjust professional behaviors
➡ Seek feedback
➡ Manage time effectively
➡ Arrange cognitive and affective supports
➡ Follow through on recommendations
➡ Remember safety first
➡ Take responsibility for behaviors

Supervisor:
➡ Increase feedback and/or supervision
➡ Probe during treatment and fill in gaps in thinking
➡ Remind student of policies or procedures
➡ Contact AFWC
➡ Arrange for professional development opportunities

AFWC:
➡ Refer student to campus supports
➡ Counsel student on educational issues
➡ Arrange tutoring
➡ Coach or arrange small group discussions
➡ Monitor progress

ance. The student is protected by law. The AFWC cannot share this knowledge with the fieldwork site without the student's permission. Whatever the reasons for a student not meeting expectations, the supervisor can find support in terminating a failing student from the school's AFWC, the program's behavioral objectives, and the FWE evaluation form.

Preventing a Student from Failing

Often, the supervisor reports to the AFWC that he or she had a "funny feeling" early on in the fieldwork experience that there may be problems. Failing fieldwork students often begin to show issues at what AFWCs call *the end of the honeymoon period.* This is typically at the end of the orientation and observation period when student demands begin to increase. As soon as students seem to be behind expectations, the fieldwork supervisor should contact the AFWC. Because prevention of further problems is easier than fixing existing problems, the AFWC can assist the facility in establishing a learning contract that clearly outlines what the student needs to do to get back on track. *Learning Contract Options* suggests methods that might be included in a learning contract. School and facility resources can be put in place, and the student will understand what the consequences are of not

meeting the learning contract. If the issues are simply performance and practice, the supervisor can consider extending the length of the fieldwork experience. The AFWC can closely monitor the student's progress, providing additional support and referral as needed.

Failing a Fieldwork Student

Although schools have aggressive professional development programs in place to prevent unsuccessful students from failing on level II fieldwork, schools do expect students to fail. A highly emotional experience for all involved, the task should be based on documented behaviors evaluated by the facility's student objectives and the FWE. Documentation of specific behaviors assists the student in taking responsibility and helps the school put in place an effective remediation plan. Documentation of specific behaviors further helps the fieldwork supervisor remain in the "educator" role instead of the more comfortable "therapist" role. The AFWC should be involved prior to the final evaluation and can provide support to both the student and the supervisor. A final meeting of the student, the supervisor, and the AFWC helps bring closure to the experience and assists the student in leaving with a positive moment. After the meeting, be sure to return all appropriate forms and evaluations to the school as soon as possible. This will assist the AFWC in developing a plan for the future with the student.

Remediation Plan

Following a fieldwork termination, the school will assist the student in developing an action plan. Highly individualized and often including educational counseling, the AFWC will suggest remediation specific to the issues the student showed during fieldwork. Once the plan has been completed and the school is satisfied with the student's progress, another fieldwork placement might be arranged. The student may or may not allow the AFWC to disclose to the potential site that this is a repeat fieldwork, although the AFWC will likely encourage the student to disclose special supervision methods needed. The AFWC, aware of earlier problems, will likely follow this fieldwork closely.

SUMMARY

This chapter outlined how to develop a fieldwork program for your facility. Myths and arguments against fieldwork were dispelled. An outline was presented to help organize the fieldwork development process. Cognitive and affective factors related to the failing student were addressed.

REFERENCES

Adelstein, L. A., Cohn, E. S., Baker, R. C., & Barnes, M. A. (1990). A part-time level II fieldwork program. *Am J Occup Ther, 44*(1), 60-65.

Accreditation Council for Occupational Therapy Education. (1998a). *Standards for an accredited educational program for the occupational therapist*. Bethesda, MD: American Occupational Therapy Association.

Accreditation Council for Occupational Therapy Education. (1998b). *Standards for an accredited educational program for the occupational therapist assistant*. Bethesda, MD: American Occupational Therapy Association.

Atwater, A., & Davis, C. (1990). The value of psychosocial level II fieldwork. *Am J Occup Ther, 44*(9), 792-795.

Bloomer, J. (1995). Applied research during fieldwork: Interdisciplinary collaboration between universities and clinics. *Am J Occup Ther, 49*, 207-213.

Declute, J., & Ladyshewsky, R. (1993). Enhancing clinical competence using a collaborative clinical education model. *Phys Ther, 73*(10), 683-689.

Gutman, S., McCreedy, P., & Heisler, P. (1998). Student level II fieldwork failure: Strategies for intervention. *Am J Occup Ther, 52*(2), 143-149.

Hengel, J. L., & Romeo, J. L. (1995). A group approach to mental health fieldwork. *Am J Occup Ther, 49*, 354-358.

Hischmann, C. (1990). Recruitment and retention in state psychiatric hospital. *Mental Health Special Interest Section Newsletter, 13*, 2-3.

Kautzmann, L. (1987). Perceptions of the purpose of level I fieldwork. *Am J Occup Ther, 41*(9), 595-560.

Lyons, M., & Ziviani, J. (1995). Stereotypes, stigma, and mental illness: Learning from fieldwork experiences. *Am J Occup Ther, 47*(6), 1002-1008.

Merrill, S., & Crist, P. (2000). *Meeting the fieldwork challenge: A self-paced clinical course from AOTA*. Bethesda, MD: American Occupational Therapy Association.

Meyers, S. (1995). Exploring the cost and benefit drives of clinical education. *Am J Occup Ther, 49*(2), 107-111.

Shalik, L. (1987). Cost-benefit analysis of level II fieldwork in occupational therapy. *Am J Occup Ther, 41*(10), 638-645.

Shalik, H., & Shalik, L. (1988). The occupational therapy level II fieldwork experience: Estimation of the fiscal benefit. *Am J Occup Ther, 42*(3), 164-168.

Siebert, C. (1997). A description of fieldwork in the home care setting. *Am J Occup Ther, 51*(6), 423-429.

Sladyk, K., & Sheckley, B. (2000). Clinical reasoning and reflective practice. *Occupational Therapy in Health Care, 13*(1), 11-22.

Swinehart, S., & Meyers, S. (1992). Level I fieldwork: Creating a positive experience. *Am J Occup Ther, 47*(1), 68-73.

Tompson, M., & Ryan, A. (1996). The influence of fieldwork on the professional socialization of occupational therapy students. *British Journal of Occupational Therapy, 58*, 65-70.

Walker, E. M. (1995). Improving the links: Fieldwork educators' conferences. *British Journal of Therapy and Rehabilitation, 2*, 382-385.

Appendix A

IMPORTANT CONTACT INFORMATION

ACADEMIC FIELDWORK COORDINATOR

Name

AFWC Office Phone Number

AFWC Email Address

School OT Office Phone Number

School FAX Number

Home Phone Number

Home Email Address

Cell Phone (if available)

Other Numbers

Please limit phone calls to home (or cell) phone to the following hours:

PROGRAM DIRECTOR OR OTHER EMERGENCY COVERAGE PERSON

Name

Office Phone Number

Home Phone Number

FIELDWORK EDUCATOR

Name, Address, Office Phone Number, Email Address for Each Site

Appendix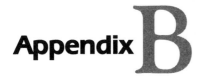

INTERNET RESOURCES

As I said in *Ryan's Occupational Therapy Assistant* (Ryan & Sladyk, 2000), trying to keep an internet resource list current is like trying to hold water in your hands, but these sites are good places to start. Each site has been reviewed for accurate contact and has been judged as stable. The reader is cautioned to evaluate internet information with extreme care. Because internet information is not peer reviewed and the author is often unknown, the worth of internet material is often of no scientific value. Internet information is fast, but students are cautioned that the internet does not replace scholarly inquiry.

To evaluate a web site, look for content accuracy first. Does the site publish information that you know is true from other reliable print forms such as journals? What seems to be the mission of the web site? Are they trying to sell you something? Are they fundraising for their cause? Both sales and fundraising are acceptable internet tools, but does that seem to be the main purpose of a national organization's web site? Are authors' names and peer reviewed material available on the site?

Formats that are user friendly and accessible make a web site easier to use but do not be mislead by slick web sites that lack scientific content. Reliable sites have web masters that can accurately blend content and ease of use. The bottom line: Be very, very careful of internet information and make sure you confirm all content with noninternet resources.

SITE THAT PROVIDES LINKS TO OTHER OCCUPATIONAL THERAPY SITES

Occupational Therapy
www.occupationaltherapist.com

SITES OF INTEREST TO OCCUPATIONAL THERAPY FIELDWORK STUDENTS

Administration on Aging
www.aoa.dhhs.gov

Advance for Occupational Therapy Practitioners
www.advanceforot.com

Alzheimer's Association
www.alz.org

American Association of Retired Persons
www.aarp.org

American Cancer Society
www.cancer.org

American Diabetes Association
www.diabetes.org/custom.asp

American Dietetic Association
www.eatright.org

American Occupational Therapy Association
www.aota.org

American Occupational Therapy Foundation
www.aotf.org

Arthritis Foundation
www.arthritis.org

Bartleby Desk References
www.bartleby.com/reference

Centers for Medicare & Medicaid Services
www.hcfa.gov

CINAHL
www.cinahl.com

CNN Health
www.cnn.com/health

Community Access Program (CAP)
www.hrsa.dhhs.gov/CAP

Department of Veterans Affairs
www.va.gov

Discovery Channel
www.discovery.com

Elderhostel
www.elderhostel.org

Find Tutorials
www.findtutorials.com

Grants Network
www.hhs.gov/grantsnet

Health on the Net Foundation
www.hon.ch

Health Finder
www.healthfinder.gov

Health Web
www.healthweb.org

HumorMatters
www.humormatters.com

ICIDH-2
www.who.int/icidh

Juvenile Diabetes Research Foundation International
www.jdfcure.org

Leisure and Aging Center
http://web.indstate.edu/nrpa-las/links.html

Medicare
www.medicare.gov

Muscle Charts of the Human Body
www.ptcentral.com/muscles

Muscular Dystrophy Association
www.mdausa.org

National Board for Certification in Occupational Therapy
www.nbcot.org

National Cancer Institute
www.nci.nih.gov

National Council on the Aging
www.ncoa.org

National Eye Institute
www.nei.nih.gov

National Institute of Arthritis and Musculoskeletal and Skin Diseases
www.niams.nih.gov

National Institute of Child Health & Human Development
www.nichd.nih.gov

National Institute of Diabetes & Digestive & Kidney Diseases
www.niddk.nih.gov

National Institutes of Health
www.nih.gov

National Institute of Mental Health
www.nimh.nih.gov

National Institute of Neurological Disorders and Stroke
www.ninds.nih.gov

National Institute on Aging
www.nia.nih.gov

National Institute on Alcohol Abuse and Alcoholism
www.niaaa.nih.gov

National Institute on Deafness and Other Communication Disorders
www.nidcd.nih.gov

National Institute on Drug Abuse
www.nida.nih.gov

National Library of Medicine
www.nlm.nih.gov

National Mental Health Association
www.nmha.org

National Osteoporosis Foundation
www.nof.org

National Parkinson Foundation
www.parkinson.org

National Rehabilitation Information Center
www.naric.com

National Stroke Association
www.stroke.org

Prevent Blindness America
www.preventblindness.org

Social Security
www.ssa.gov

US Department of Health & Human Services
www.hhs.gov

US Food and Drug Administration
www.fda.gov

US Government Guidelines on Evidence-Based Practice (Agency for Healthcare Research and Quality)
www.ahrq.gov

World Federation of Occupational Therapists
www.who.int/ina-ngo/ngo/ngo170.htm

World Health Organization
www.who.int

REFERENCE

Ryan, S. E., & Sladyk, K. (2000). *Ryan's occupational therapy assistant: Principles, practice issues, and techniques* (3rd ed.). Thorofare, NJ: SLACK Incorporated.

INDEX